W9-APM-905

Hello Beautiful

Published by MQ Publications Limited
12 The Ivories, 6–8 Northampton Street, London N1 2HY
Tel: 020 7359 2244 / Fax: 020 7359 1616
email: mail@mqpublications.com

Copyright © Susie Galvez 2003
Published under exclusive license by MQ Publications Ltd
The moral rights of the author have been asserted

Design: Dennis Michael Stredney

ISBN: 1-84072-443-9

1 3 5 7 9 0 8 6 4 2

All rights reserved. No part of this publication may be reproduced or transmitted in any form or by any means, electronic or mechanical, including photocopy, recording, or any information storage and retrieval system now known or to be invented without permission in writing from the publishers.

Printed and bound in China

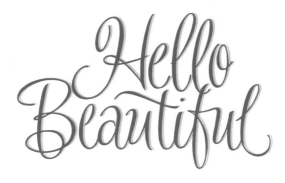

Hello Beautiful

365 ways to be even more beautiful

Susie Galvez

MQP

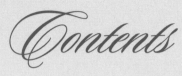

Contents

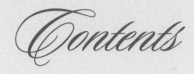

Contents

Introduction

"To wash one's hair, make one's toilet, and put on scented robes; even if not a soul sees one, these preparations still produce an inner pleasure."
Sei Shonagon

My fascination with beauty products and techniques probably began subconsciously around the age of five. Watching my mother at her dressing table amid all of the beautiful bottles and jars of wonderfully scented lotions and creams allowed me to witness the art of beauty, and I have been forever captivated.

Over the years, my observations became more formal as a student and later professional in the beauty industry. As an esthetician, makeup artist, and day spa owner, I have the privilege of teaching what I have learned to individuals on a daily basis, but this book allows me to reach a much larger audience. *Hello Beautiful* provides me the opportunity to share with you the head to toe tips and techniques I have learned from experience and hard work.

Most importantly, never forget that true beauty is more than applying makeup and spritzing on fragrance. Beauty is an internal factor that is apparent in individuals who are comfortable and confident in their own skin.

It is my sincerest hope that you enjoy reading *Hello Beautiful* as much as I enjoyed writing it for you.

Susie Galvez

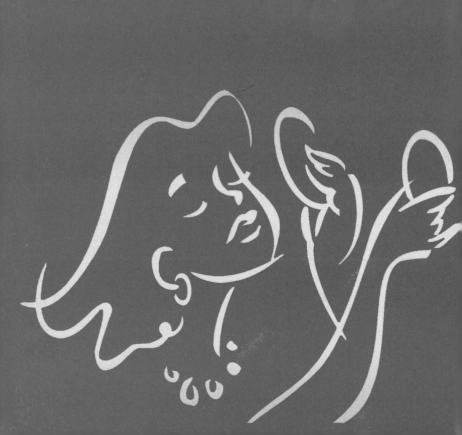

Chapter 1

Saving Face

"In the factory we make cosmetics; in the store we sell hope."
Charles Revson

While a true miracle in a jar has yet to be invented, good skin care offers the best insurance against wrinkles, lines, puffiness, spots, and discolorations. A beauty routine of **2-3 MINUTES** in the **AM** and **PM** is all that you need to keep your skin looking its best.

1 Tone Up

Not using a toner/skin freshener after you cleanse your skin is like putting your washed clothes into the dryer without using the rinse cycle. The toner/freshener **helps remove any cleanser and debris** as well as helping the skin return to a **normal ph balance.**

Bosom Buddies

The skin on the *décolleté* (neck and chest area) is very sensitive and has no fat tissue. This area shows the telltale signs of aging such as sunspots, wrinkling, and dryness. Instead of using soap to clean this delicate area, use your facial cleansing cream. Creams that are designed for your face will hydrate while gently cleansing. Finish with your facial moisture cream.

3

Hide Out

When applying sunscreen, don't forget the back of the neck, the hairline, and especially the ears. Also always rub the extra on the back of your hands—*liver spots will never be in style!*

Fab Beauty
FLASH

Need to look rested and fabulous in 15 minutes or less? Apply a hydrating creamy mask on the face and neck. Put a **slice of cucumber** on the closed eyelids. Lie down and rest for 10 minutes. Remove the cucumber slices and for the next five minutes hang your head off the side of the bed allowing the blood to circulate. After you rinse and hydrate with your favorite moisturizer, you will feel like a new person—*ready for anything!*

2 X 30 (31) = Beautiful Skin

A skincare regime used twice a day will produce superior results compared to anything a professional spa can do on even a once a month basis. Properly cleansing, toning, exfoliating, and hydrating twice daily combined with regularly scheduled spa visits, will produce the best skin possible for you.

2X

6

Steam It Up

Concoct a pore cleaning, refreshing herbal

steam bath for the face.

Boil a large pot of water. Remove from heat, stir in 2 tablespoons of some herbs from your health food store and let them steep for 5 minutes. Place a towel over your head and let steam bathe your face for 3 to 5 minutes, while turning your face to reach all sides. Rinse with cool water, then hydrate. Skin and pores will be clean and healthy.

PRO KNOWS

7

X4

For the absolute best skin possible, try to have a professional facial treatment at the very least four times a year. Having professional facials is like 'spring cleaning' for the face.

Frequent Flier Miles

Anyone who frequently flies knows what a number the **DRY, RE-CIRCULATED AIR ON PLANES** can do to the skin. Carry a small mister bottle of mineral water and spritz yourself whenever you start to feel dry. Also, remember to drink plenty of water and curb the caffeine and alcohol which are both dehydrating.

9

Play Misty for Me

Spritzing your face after cleansing but before moisturizing will **plump up** your skin locking in moisture for up to *12 hours.*

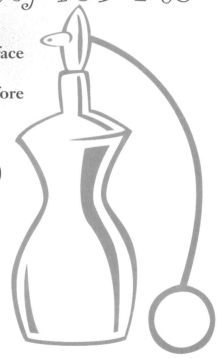

Just Say NO

THere is no safe tan.

Applying a topical vitamin C cream with a sun block cream increases its effectiveness against skin damage, dehydration, and wrinkles. If you are sensitive to chemical sunscreens try ones containing titanium dioxide as a base. Titanium dioxide is a natural mineral that acts as a physical block to UVA and UVB rays.

Lip Polish

To keep lips their softest, *kissable best,* use a lip exfoliator once or twice a week. The mild pumice granules will remove old cakey lip color and excess dead skin. Rinse and re-hydrate with a vitamin C and E stick.

Picky, Picky, Picky

Resist the temptation to pick or squeeze the skin.

Skin scars very easily.

Leave the deep cleaning facials and blackhead

extraction to the experts. Quit the assault.

Loosen up

If after you have cleansed and toned your skin, your skin feels tight and squeaky clean—you probably have just shrunk it. The taut feeling is caused by the removal of all hydration thus causing the skin to shrink. Switch to a cleanser and toner that cleanses without stripping the skin. You want to be able to smile without

'CRACKING UP!'

Warm Hands

To get the most from skincare treatment products, rub them in your hands before applying. This will produce a **warming effect** and make the product easier to spread.

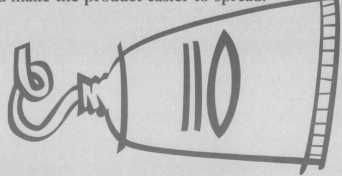

15

keepIt **Up**

Gravity pulls the skin down, so when applying treatment products work up and out toward the forehead and hairline. Do what the professionals do and lightly pat the products on with your fingertips in **circular motions,** which will increase circulation.

WAIT A MINUTE

Better yet **wait a few minutes** after applying hydrating products to the skin before starting your makeup. If the product does not have time to penetrate, when makeup is applied, it can cause smearing and spotty applications.

Lucky Number 13

The skin renews itself about **13** times a year. Over the course of a lifetime, more than **30** pounds of dead skin cells will be shed. In fact, over **80** percent of dust is shed skin cells! Hard on the dust cloth, but good for your skin.

18 OpenWide

When visiting the **Dentist,** take along a

moisturizing lip balm. Apply to the lips to keep

them

from

cracking.

NATURAL IS **NOT** ALWAYS BETTER

Poison Ivy is natural, but you would not put it on your face. Chemicals can help products last longer, keep them bacteria free, and aid in further penetration of 'natural' ingredients.

Science and nature need to work in harmony.

Out with the OLD

Sunscreen's active ingredients typically have a **2-year** shelf life. Date yours when you open it, and throw it out in **2** years or sooner if it starts to change color, separate, or smell funny. After all, you only have one skin—treat it right.

To Tell the Truth

Remove all of those over-promised and under-delivered creams and potions from your facial regime. Relegate them to be used up via body and foot creams. And then make a promise to *only buy products that really work!*

White Wash

Schedule a teeth-whitening session with your dentist. It is one of the most effective and affordable ways to brighten your face.

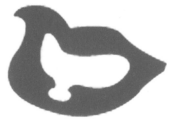

GETTING READY TO
Get Ready

Getting ready to go out should be as much **fun** as actually going out. Put some great **music** on while you makeup. **Dance around** while you dress. You will go out feeling great and the feeling will last all evening.

You Got the TOUCH

By touching your skin via cleansing, exfoliating, hydrating, and the like you are stimulating circulation and facilitating the removal of toxins and absorption of nutrients. **The more you *touch* your skin, the more *touchable* it becomes.**

Vogue

Beautiful handbag. Fantastic shoes. Incredible designer clothes. All of them will never cover up neglected skin. Did you know that some people take better care of a silk blouse than they do of their skin? Enjoy the couture, but take care of your skin.

FACE IT

Remember at **20** years old, you have the face that God gave you, at **40** you have the face you have purchased, and at **60** you have the face you deserve. So start as young as you are and go as long as you're alive. Don't be the one who wakes up at fifty-something and says: "Wow, I should have worn an eye cream!"

27
Put Your Feet **Up**

To get the best results from a facial mask, put your feet up. Blood-circulating oxygen is then redirected from the lower body to the head, allowing for better absorption of mask ingredients. Besides helping your facial skin, **relaxing your feet** for 10–15 minutes **is relaxing for the entire body** Prop 'em up for a few.

Save Face

When trying new products, **try them at night.**
That way if you have a reaction, you have several
hours for the skin to recoup. You don't want to
apply a disagreeable facial mask one hour before
a big meeting or first date. Yikes!

Extraction
Attraction

Remove blackheads by combining ¼ cup of very hot water and 1 teaspoon of Epsom salts with 4 drops of iodine. Mix well and let cool until just slightly warm to the touch. Dip a cotton ball or swab and apply to blackhead and surrounding area. Wait for mixture to dry and then gently remove with a washcloth. Repeat if necessary. *Note: Do not force blackheads out by squeezing them —it will cause permanent scaring.*

30 Puff in Stuff

Under eye puffiness is simply water retention. To encourage fluids to be reabsorbed into the body, let gravity take its course by moving. KEEP MOVING—take a walk, do some housework—just move it. The sooner you get moving, the sooner those pesky bags will hit the road.

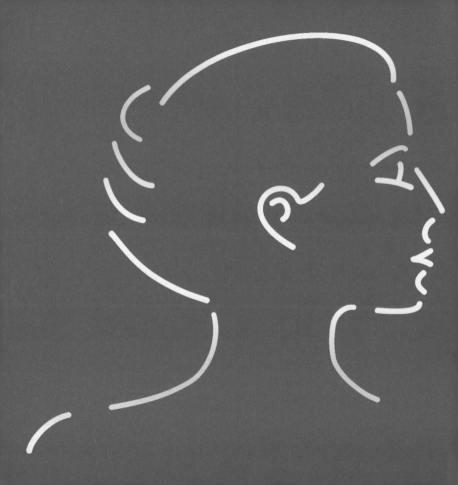

Chapter 2

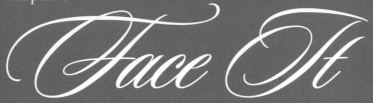

Face It

"Lots of women buy just as many makeup things as I do. They just don't wear them all at the same time."

Dolly Parton

akeup is a tool to help you look your best. Think of makeup as an accessory to **showcase your assets.** Cosmetics should be used to enhance, not disguise your unique features. A little blush here, a dab of gloss there and suddenly you are ready to greet the world with confidence.

31

GOT CHA' COVERED

Even if your foundation contains sunscreen, it is best to still *wear sun protection* underneath because makeup tends to migrate toward the lines and wrinkles throughout the day leaving some skin unprotected.

It's All In The Wrist

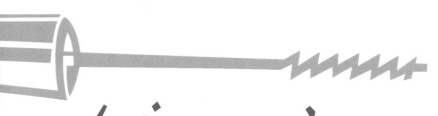

If you **'zigzag'** the wand while applying mascara, you will help separate and color each lash. This also reduces clumping.

33

TWO IS BETTER THAN ONE

Always apply *two coats of mascara*—

one for **color** and the second to add

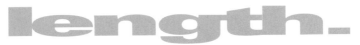

34

Brush Up

A professional set of COSMETIC BRUSHES is a gal's best friend. The correct tools allow for the perfect makeup application each and every time.

Clean As A Whistle

Clean professional cosmetic brushes and applicators in anti-bacterial soap at least **once a month**, rinse, put bristles in original brush shape and let air-dry. Keep makeup build up and bacteria at bay.

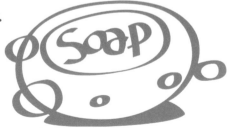

BROW-Zing!

A good eyebrow will perfectly frame the face. Well-shaped brows make the eyes look bigger and cheekbones look higher. It is worth the cost of having a brow designing session with a professional. The session will provide brow shaping and teach you how to take care of your brows and maintain their perfect shape.

Make It Believable

Blending two or three brow colors will create the most natural look. Our hair is more than one color, so are our brows. Apply the brow color by starting at the outside of the brow rather than from the inside. By going backwards into brow hair using short strokes, you will help fill in where you may need color or to give the look of more brow hairs. Then using a brow brush, brush the brows back into place. Brows will look natural yet full.

BRONZE MEDAL

Bronzing powders are wonderful for helping to create the monochromatic look. Use it to shadow eyes, as a finishing powder for lips, to soften eyebrows, and as a finishing powder to set makeup.

sun-kissed

Sweep a big powder brush of bronzer across the cheeks and nose. This will create the sun-kissed look of the tropics without the sun damage.

Kiss Me Quick

Lipstick protects the lips from all sorts of environmental damage and keeps the lips from chapping. Plus, as an extra bonus, studies show that *lipstick wearers kiss,* on average, **60 times a week** as compared to **20 times** for bare-lippers!

Take the
TINT

Tinted eyebrows and eyelashes make getting ready in the morning a snap since you can skip the brow and lash coloring. The tint lasts about four weeks, and as an added bonus, you will look good even before you get out of bed!

connect the dots

Apply foundation by dotting the face with 5-6 dots of foundation.

Apply with a cosmetic sponge to forehead, cheeks, nose, and chin. Blend lightly, using your sponge for a flawless finish. Be sure to blend downward to prevent de-markation lines near chin and neck and to make the little facial hairs lay down.

Prime Time

Applying a small

dab of eye shadow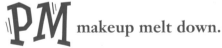

primer to each eyelid will help keep eye shadow

hours longer than the usual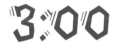

PM makeup melt down.

44

TAKE A POWDER

After applying foundation lightly dust finishing

powder all over the face. Powder sets your makeup

the same way hair spray sets your hair!

Line 'em Up

Lip liner following the natural contours of the lip area will keep lip color from straying up into the tiny pucker lines. Coloring in the entire lip with liner before applying lipstick will help keep lip color on longer. A perfect remedy for when you can't refreshen right away.

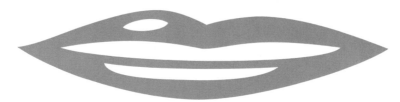

A Little **DAB** Will Do Ya

Put a little eye cream above the lip area to

help firm and fight wrinkles. It also helps control

lipstick bleed.

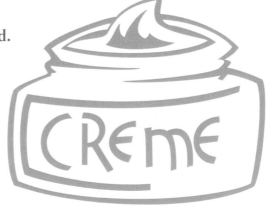

Curl up

Use an eyelash curler to open your eyes and create the thickest, longest lashes possible. **Never curl lashes with mascara on,** this will cause them to break or fall out. Place the base of the curler right up to the upper eyelid and gently press closed. Hold for a count of at least 10. Gently open and repeat on the other eye. You will see lashes you didn't even know you had! Add your favorite colored mascara and wow!

Get Cheeky

To make blush last its longest, use a tiny bit of cream blush first, powder the face, and then add powder blush. **The blush will last as long as you do!** By placing the powder blush over a powdered face, you will not experience blotchiness that can occur when blush is applied directly to the skin.

YOU'RE BLUSHING

For the most natural blush color, check the color of your lips when you're not wearing lipstick. Your natural lip pigment is the perfect color for your blush. Another good way to select the right blush color is to look at your cheeks after you have been exerting yourself slightly.

ATTENTION GETTER

Place a small (about the size of a dime) dot of a golden or light reflecting color of eye shadow on the center of your eyelid, then blend slightly. When you are blinking, people will notice the light area but won't know why. Humans are naturally attracted to the light. Try it and see if you don't have more **eye contact** during the day!

Luscious Lips

Dab a dot of shiny lip gloss in the center of the

bottom lip. As it catches the light, so will you.

Lipstick teeth—NO WAY

A makeup artist trick is to put your index finger in your mouth, close your lips around it and pull your finger out. Any excess lipstick will stick to the skin on your finger and not to your teeth.

Turn OFF the WATER-PROOF

Waterproof mascara is too harsh on the lashes. It coats the lash and as it dries it shrinks around the lash body. This shrinking can cause breakage and lash fall out. Also waterproof is harder to remove resulting in more rubbing of the eye area. **Stick to water-resistant which is much easier on the eyes.**

54
YOU'RE OUT!

Clean out your makeup drawer

ridding it of all the half-used, broken, held together with a rubber band products that you haven't used in a year. Don't feel guilty—your beauty drawer is not a time capsule for future generations. **GIVE IT THE HEAVE HO.**

Head Over Heels

One way to find exactly where your blush should go is to **bend over and touch the floor** for a few seconds. When you stand back up, you'll see exactly where you are flushed and that's where the blush should go. Perfect every time.

In the Shadows

Blush can work beautifully as eye shadow

if the blush color is natural looking (not too pink). Blend it lightly over the entire lid, eyes will look lovely and your eye color will really stand out.

See the Light

Proper makeup application requires proper lighting. You don't get dressed in the dark, and you shouldn't apply your face there. Change the bulbs to **60** watts at least or **25** watts if makeup mirror light is used.

By the Light of Day

Give your makeup the light test.

After you've finished your makeup application, check out your work in a hand mirror by a bright daylight window. If you pass the sunlight test which means no streaks, smears, or unblended anything, then your application is perfect!

59
ARRIVE IN FIVE

If you only have **5** minutes to apply your makeup—use the **'kiss'** method *(keep it super simple)*. Use one-color or monochromatic makeup to create harmony when in a rush. Bronzy or delicate pinks are perfect and give a finished look on the go. **So get going!**

Splurge
Buy a new lipstick.

Pick a *'pick-me-up'* color and splurge! To test colors put some lipstick on inside of the fingertips instead of on the back of your hand. The color on the inside of your fingertips is the most like the lips, and will give you a better idea of how the color will look on your lips. Now that's true beauty at your fingertips!

Lip Service

In a pinch, lipstick can 'do' as a blush or eyeshadow if blended correctly. But due to the waxes in lipstick, it should not be used on an ongoing basis. But it sure works well if it's all you have at the moment!

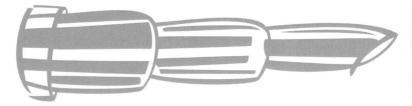

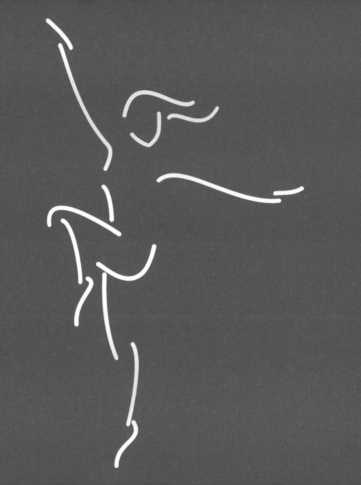

Chapter 3

Body Beautiful

"The finest clothing made is a person's own skin."
Mark Twain

Handle your body with care. Indulging and pampering yourself is an indication of self-respect. If you feel good in your skin—it shows—in how you stand, move, and touch others.

BRUSH UP

Dry brushing the skin is a wonderful technique for improving skin tone, circulation, and for helping the skin rid itself of dry, dead skin cells. Start at the feet and move the brush in long, gentle strokes in an upward motion, always going towards the heart. Continue with legs, thighs, abdomen, stomach, arms, and back. Shower, dry, and apply hydration. About once a week wash your brush with soap and water to keep it free of skin debris.

Shine On

Open the curtains and let the sunshine in. Bright natural light early in the day enhances the body's internal rhythms and helps you sleep better at night.

SHRUG IT OFF

Shoulder shrugs are easy stretches that release tension from the upper body. Shrug off the day before retiring by inhaling and tightening your shoulders, pulling them up towards your ears. Exhale while gently relaxing your shoulders. Repeat three times.

A-H-H-H-H-H!

SWEET DREAMS

The deep, **sweet scent of vanilla** summons a sense of calm. While changing clothes for bed, light a vanilla candle. Moisturize hands and arms with a vanilla scented cream. Tension will be extracted.

Good night!

Scent-sational Idea!

TRY A NEW SCENT AND LAYER IT.

Start with a bath or shower gel, then body crème,

dusting powder, and perfume. Remember behind

the knees as well as the pulse points for the

longest lasting aroma.

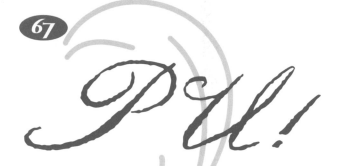

PU!

Accidentally spritzed *too much perfume,* or tried a sample that turned stinky? Take a warm soapy washcloth and gently cleanse pulse points, or wherever the fragrance was applied. Rinse with cool water and blot dry.

Get a Leg Up

Legs have very few oil glands and are subject to dryness and flaky skin. Hosiery can actually accelerate the condition acting like a cheese grater on the legs. Remember to **slather the legs with body cream before putting on clothing—** especially hosiery.

69
Get Moving

Nothing helps circulate the blood more than moving. Yoga, dancing, walking, running, even pacing while on the telephone gets the blood pumping. **REMEMBER, MOVE IT OR LOSE IT.**

Sachet Fancy

Tuck a lavender sachet under your pillow before leaving for the day. When you come home and are ready to retire, you will sleep better, and everything will smell clean, fresh, and summery. pleasant dreams.

Bare Footing

Workout barefoot occasionally to strengthen the small muscles in the foot. This method is especially good for yoga, stretching, and pilates.

72

SHHHH!

Never interrupt when you are being flattered.
Allow the compliment to swirl around like fine
wine on your tongue, through your ears. Wait a
moment, and then sincerely say "Thank you."

Enjoy the moment!

Gimme Me **TWO**

Two minutes of teeth brushing is necessary twice a day to really get the teeth their cleanest. Most people brush for 30 seconds! Get a timer and set it for 2 minutes—if it seems like an eternity— think about all of the things you were missing in your mouth before now!

take a deep breath

Bad breath is a beauty breaker.

A sure way to see if you need a breath mint ASAP is to lick your palm and smell it while it's still wet. If it is less than fresh, you can count on bad breath. Pop a mint quick! Your public will thank you!

Seeing Spots

Avoid wearing perfumes, or scented lotions when out in the sun. These products can cause the skin to blotch when exposed to the sun. Spots look good on animals—but not the human kind.

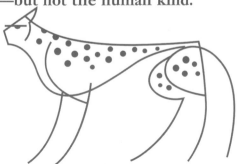

TAKE FIVE

If you're having trouble sleeping, one or two of these ideas are sure to give you the **Z-Z-Z-ZS.** Establish a regular lights out time and stick to it. Keep your sleeping area dark. This tells your body that it is time to relax and go to sleep. Sleep on soft, lightweight sheets and a lightweight blanket instead of yards of heavy covers. Set your bedroom temperature at the ideal night-time temperature of 60–65 °F (15.5-18°C) for optimum relaxation. Taking a warm bath within two hours of going to bed is another way to catch a few extra winks.

EXPOSE *yourself*

Sometimes the only skin that gets care is the skin that shows, for example face and hands. **Skin on the body is often neglected.** Putting body lotion on twice a day takes less than 5 minutes. Exfoliating with a body scrub in the shower is something that can be done while the hair is conditioning. *Remember it is skin—* **not cotton** *—that is the fabric of our lives.*

GOT THE ITCH

Scratch a small area on your leg with your fingernail. If this leaves a jet stream-like line on the leg, your skin is covered with dead, dry skin. **It is time to exfoliate by either dry brushing, and/or using scrubs in the shower**. Be sure to hydrate afterwards.

Honey Do

Honey is a natural humectant (holds moisture) as well as a natural antibacterial, so it is perfect as an ingredient in body or face products. Internally, it works the same way. So if it is good enough for the Queen Bee, it should be good enough for you. *Be a honey to yourself and put a little honey in your life.*

Foot Loose

Always remember to apply sunscreen on the top of the feet including the toes before going out in the sun. It is the most forgotten part of the body to sunscreen. The sun beats down right on top of the toes and feet, so protect those footsies!

Bee's Knees

Knees can age you close up and from a distance.

Dry brush, exfoliate, and keep them hydrated at all times. You can get down on your knees, but keep up with their care!

in Touch

Having a professional massage is not only de-stressing and relaxing, but a full body massage is also wonderful for stimulating circulation, allowing blood to flow more freely through the entire body from the top of the head to the tip of toes. Blood pressure can be lowered, and with increased circulation, your brain is more alert. Endorphins are increased, easing depression and inspiring an overall feeling of well-being. ALL YOU HAVE TO DO IS LIE DOWN, AND LET THE MASSAGE THERAPIST'S GIFTED HANDS DO THE REST.

UN-DO the OVERDO

If you are still insisting on getting in the sun, and by chance overdo it, a sunburn can be soothed by soaking in a tub of lukewarm water with an entire box of baking soda sprinkled in it.

(Obviously, the smartest thing is to avoid the sunburn altogether!)

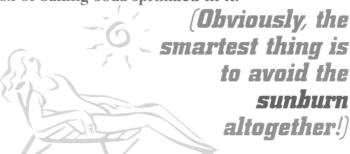

Bird Bath

When you have **no time to shower,** put a sponge or washcloth in a sink that is half-filled with water and several tablespoons of baking soda. Squeeze out the excess water and wipe yourself down for a good freshener. Great idea for a fast transition from work to evening out.

ANIMAL INSTINCT

Take a tip from the animal kingdom.

Before rising and before exercising, gently stretch the muscles and yawn deeply. Both movements will invigorate as well as help loosen up joints and muscles to avoid injury during exercise. Plus it feels truly wonderful all over! So **s-t-r-e-t-c-h i-t!!!**

Lose Five Pounds—Instantly!

All you have to do is stand up straight.

Drooping bodies with hunched shoulders make you look heavier and older. Every time you catch sight of yourself slumping over, remind yourself that good posture is good for your looks and great for your spine.

Free Flowing

Varicose veins can be caused by tight, constrictive clothing that restricts blood flow. This includes girdles, garters, overly zealous pantyhose, hosiery with restrictive bands, tight knee socks, and pinching waistbands on skirts or pants. **Wear properly fitted garments—always—**it will protect those beautiful gams and loosen up that 'I feel awful' look on your face caused by clothes that are too tight!

Support Your Local Stocking

Support hose protect the leg wall and help with vein circulation.

These stockings are especially good for those who sit or stand for long periods at a time. Plus with modern technology, you no longer look like your grandmother, or the old lady down the street.

The Bottom Line

To firm your 'bottom line' try tensing the 'bum' muscles while you are sitting down.

Squeeze the muscles as if you are trying to hold a pencil between your buttocks and then relax. Repeat **10** times. Another good butt burner is to lie on your back on the floor. Place your feet in a chair. Press your heels as hard as you can in the chair without lifting your bottom from the floor. Repeat **10** times. Burn, body, burn.

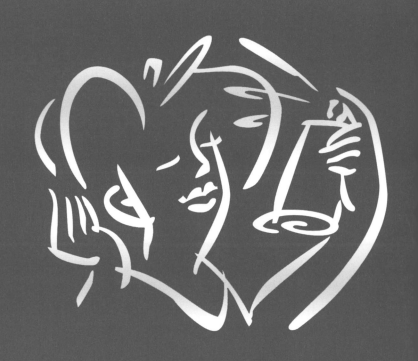

Chapter 4

Mane Event

"Another thing about women is that they can be persuaded to do anything with their hair, except leave it alone."
Unknown

We shampoo, blow dry, cut, color, crimp, braid, curl, style, and straighten our crowning glory on a daily basis all in the name of looking good. **How you feel about your hair can have a dramatic effect on your mood.** When it is a good hair day all is right with the world. Bad hair day... well, you know the story.

PHOTO OP

Choosing a hairstyle from a magazine or style book may not be a great idea since the person in the photograph is not you. Before choosing a style, ask yourself these questions: **"How does this style suit my face shape, hair type, or my age?" "Is this a look that I could recreate at home?"** Don't be afraid to interview hair designers before deciding who gets to create your very special personal look. It may only be hair, but the wrong style could affect your whole day... every day, until it grows out.

Do the 'Do

Choosing the right hair-care products is the most important part of being able to create the style day in and day out. If you have color you should always consider the type and condition of your hair before making a product decision. **With so many products to choose from, you can most certainly find one that meets your total needs.** If you need a shampoo that cleanses as well as enhances color, or a daily conditioner in order to be able to comb through your hair, don't compromise! After all you see your stylist once every 5–6 weeks, but you face your mirror every morning!

JUNK THE GUNK

Hair fixatives such as gels, hair sprays, and mousse cause buildups. If you use these types of products on a daily or weekly basis, **your hair will need de-gunking or cleansing to remove the buildups.** Clarifying shampoos are designed to deep clean the hair and remove any fixative buildup leaving the hair healthy and clean. Use a gentle clarifying shampoo designed for your hair type at least once a week. Your hair will thank you with great shine and luster.

93

Cool It!

Blow-drying hair daily can be damaging if not done properly. The damage occurs when your hair is between the damp and the dry stage. **When you feel your hair start to become dry, switch the blow dryer to a cool setting.** Stop drying all together just a tiny bit before the hair is totally dry. This will help with the dry fly-aways as well as keep the hair shiny.

LEAVE IT ON

Every other week give your hair a much needed spa session. Instead of rushing the conditioner on and off the hair, leave it on for **15–20 minutes.** Wrap the hair in a towel, sit and relax with a cup of antioxidant tea. Rinse your hair and style as usual. Your hair will feel like silk, and your scalp will be hydrated.

HAIR SPEAKS VOLUMES

In order to create beautiful hairstyles, use the products that complement your hair texture. For *fine hair:* create more volume by using hair spray, gels, and mousses. Avoid shiners and silicones as they tend to weigh fine hair down and can look greasy. **Thick hair:** styling aids that are light and liquid are best to comb through your full mane. Shine products are excellent to create a smoother, softer look. *Curly hair:* create bouncy curls with liquid stylers, light gels, or pomades. It is best to avoid mousses and thick gels. **STRAIGHT HAIR:** add extra sleekness with mousses and gels, and don't forget to add a little shine!

Color You Beautiful

Coloring your hair is a fabulous way to add a little excitement to your personal style. When choosing a color make sure it matches your skin tone. If your skin tone has a yellowish cast, you should choose colors with a golden hue or warm tone. If you are pinker in nature, ash or other cooler tones will suit you best. **ALWAYS CONSULT WITH AN EXPERT HAIR COLORIST BEFORE CHANGING.** Just because it looks good on the box, does not mean that it will look good on you. Trust me.

"Do it"

Get a new hairdo and be bold. If you are still wearing last year's hair, you need a change. Check out magazines and watch TV for a 'Do you like. But remember, your face, body, and lifestyle need to come into play when designing a total look. Depending on the style, hair is one of the fastest ways to age or de-age you.

WASH IT RIGHT OUT OF YOUR HAIR

RINSE, rinse, rinse *your hair after washing.* If smooth and silky hair is your aim, proper rinsing is crucial. Even the best conditioners will leave your hair drab and dull if not rinsed out completely.

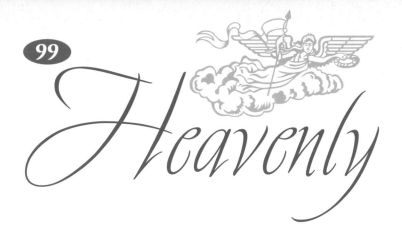

Heavenly

Next time you visit your hairstylist, ask the shampoo technician to spend extra time performing a SCALP MASSAGE. The tension will simply drain from your head, and neck. Make sure that you tip him or her appropriately for a job well done.

Less is **MORE**

To have the most silky shiny hair you may need to just leave it be. Shampoo and condition, brush, roll, and curl it less. In general treat it less. Overdoing the 'Do creates product buildup, extra tugging and pulling causes over production of sebum and that is sure to give you a dull, shine-less mane. Be kind, give it time.

You're a Natural

Dye it? Yes! Highlight it? Absolutely! But keeping your hair closer to the way it naturally grows—curly top or stick straight via no permanents or relaxers—the better your hair will look. Ringlets at the roots while the rest of your mane is board straight or dead straight roots with billowing curls is not produced in nature. Stick to creative color instead.

Bang-Bang

When trying to grow out your bangs have your stylist **add a few long layers around the face.** This will help the bangs blend in as they grow. Add a few highlights around the face to make the growing out more fun.

Scent of a Woman

For extra **PIZZAZZ** spray your hairbrush with your signature fragrance or mix a drop of fragrance with hair gel before applying to hair. As your hair moves throughout the day, your special fragrance will too.

On Best Behavior

To keep your hair on it's best behavior—*mix it up.* Switch your shampoo and conditioner every 2 or 3 weeks. When you use the same old thing all the time, your hair will start to feel weighed down, becoming difficult to style. In addition, your hair will take on a dull cast, losing its shine. *Keep it fresh.*

THE LOW DOWN

Adding a few **LOW-LIGHTS** throughout the hair creates the illusion of volume and thicker looking hair. Ask your stylist about this chic technique.

PART*ways*

zigzag

For an updated look, *zigzag* the hair's part line instead of the same old straight line. An added bonus, the crisscrossing of the part helps hide a needed color touch-up!

BED HEAD or HAT HEAD?

Fix it fast by turning your head upside down and rubbing the roots with your fingertips and combing your fingers through the hair. Spray hairspray while head is upside down. Finish by spritzing hands with hairspray and run fingers through the hair. Stand up and ta-da —like new again!

ON THE LIGHTER SIDE

Keep bangs *wispy* **and** *light*

Heavy bangs

accentuate wrinkles

and crow's feet.

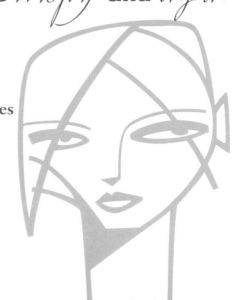

SAY HELLO TO **HIGHLIGHTS**

Highlighting the hair creates long, vertical lines and the illusion of thinness—without the diet!

A Little off the TOP

For the freshest hair, alternate your hair conditioner with one designed to remove buildup. You will feel five pounds lighter!

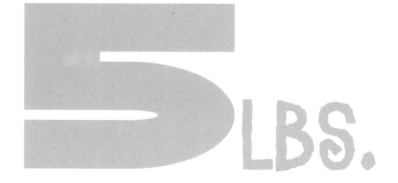

GROWDING GLORY

For an instant bit of glamour, add a FANTASTIC COLORFUL BARRETTE OR SPARKLING HAIRPINS to a sleek 'Do.

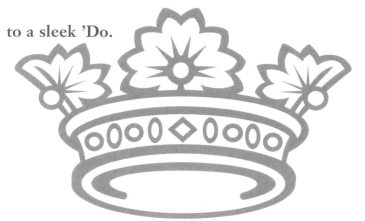

Brush Off

Take a look at your hairbrush and comb. If the bristles or teeth are worn on the ends, it's time for a new set. **Oh-h-h-h how good a new brush or comb feels to the scalp.** My-o-my, feel what you have been missing.

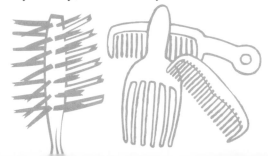

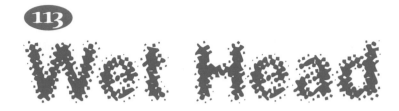

Wet Head

MAKE SURE THAT YOUR HAIR IS THOROUGHLY WET BEFORE YOU APPLY SHAMPOO. If not, the shampoo won't flow through the hair. When you try to rinse it out, some shampoo may stick to the less wet hair. The results are dull, flaky hair due to shampoo leftovers. **SO GO SOAK YOUR HEAD!**

Variety
is the Spice of Life

Next time you see your stylist ask him or her to show you **2** or **3** new ways to wear your hair and then experiment. You do not wear the same outfit everyday, **why would you have the same hairstyle day in and day out?**

Get a Good Soaking

Every month soak your hairbrush, comb, and styling accessories in hot water and some buildup removing shampoo **for 2 to 3 minutes.** Rinse and clean out hair with a comb.

In THE SWIM

Before you go in the water, slide on some conditioner to protect the hair. Afterwards rinse, rinse, rinse. A ¼ cup of apple cider mixed with ¾ of a cup of water helps rid the hair of the water from the pool or the ocean. Be sure to condition again.

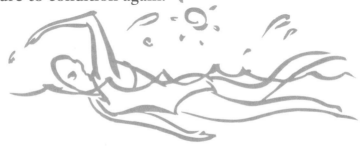

Hairdo–a Don't?

A hairstyle can nail your age in a flash. Are you wearing the same old color, length, and style of 2–5 years ago? You are not driving the same car or wearing the same clothes; why-o-why are you stuck in a time warp with your hair? update the 'Do and do it now!

HAIR Diet

There are 100s of enhancing hair products on the market. And some can actually make a difference. But the best treatment for the hair and scalp is a balanced, healthy diet. Every day is a bad hair day if your eating habits are poor.

Heads UP

Baths are wonderful for body and soul, but it is not a good idea to wash your hair in the bathtub water since body oils and dirt are released. Simply put, your hair won't get clean. Use either the shower or sink with the plug open to get the cleanest tresses.

120
Tight Rope

GO EASY ON HAIRSTYLES THAT REQUIRE YOUR HAIR BE PULLED BACK—especially if the 'Do must be tight. Stressing the hair shaft via tight buns, ponytails, or braiding can not only break the hair strand but cause trauma to the scalp resulting in damaged hair roots—permanently. Loosen up.

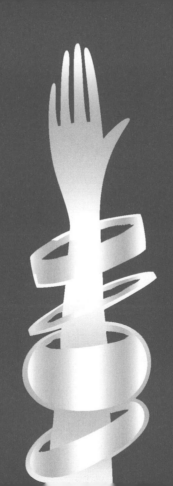

Chapter 5

Hand & Foot

"To keep your hands smooth and lovely, put two things in the dishwater—someone else's hands."
Unknown

"When a woman is dressed to kill, her feet are usually the first victims."
Unknown

Hands, nails, and feet are sure indicators of age and lifestyle. Smooth skin and manicured nails tell the world that you take yourself seriously. Whether you talk with your hands or not—they speak volumes. While your feet are usually under wraps, pampered and painted toes put a little pep in your step.

Rubbing the Right Way

Keep cuticle oil or cream at work or wherever you usually make your phone calls. While on the phone apply cuticle oil or cream and massage in. This one step will dramatically improve the entire nail area.

TOP It Off

Apply a topcoat
to a new manicure
every day.
This will keep your
nails looking great
for a week.

123

Lending a Hand

Apply hand cream before you put on rubber gloves to wash the dishes or clean.

The heat from the hot water makes the cream

5 times more effective.

WHiTE iT OuT

If your nails have white spots on them

try adding more zinc-rich foods

such as eggs, milk, or liver to your diet.

125
Fix it FAST

If you chip a nail use a file to even out edges and

apply polish only to chipped areas. Allow to dry

and add another coat of polish to the entire nail.

Magic!—chips
gone.

Wonder Where the
YELLOW Went

If your nails are discolored wet a cotton ball with

vinegar and press it to the nail for 60 seconds.

Stubborn discoloring may require a second application.

oh Darn it!

Smudged a nail?

Apply a bit of nail polish remover with the pad of

your finger to the smudged area to smooth out.

After the remover dries, add a light coat of polish.

All fixed!

Quit Picking on Me

Avoid the temptation of picking off nail polish. When you pick at the nail polish, you could pull off the top layer of the nail as well. To say nothing of what it does to your manicure.

129

Play Footsie

Place a foot roller under your foot while bearing down, roll the entire length of your foot over the tool, back and forth. Repeat, concentrating on your arches. **Do this for 5 to 10 minutes per foot.** This exercise is wonderful for relieving fatigue and cramping, especially in your arches.

ON THE BALL

Keep a golf ball in your office or beside your chair at home. While sitting, roll the golf ball under your feet for 2 minutes on each foot. **It is a tension relieving massage that helps with arch strain, foot cramps, or heel pain.** You will be refreshed and ready for anything!

Tug of War

Place a nice, thick, moderately stiff rubber band around your big toes and pull your feet away from each other slowly. Hold the **STRETCH** for **5** to **10** seconds. Repeat **10** to **20** times. This is a wonderful way to ease toe cramping or the ouch of bunions caused by wearing tight fitting shoes.

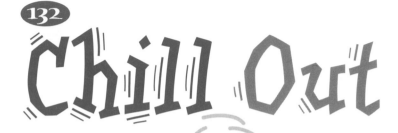

132
Chill Out

For an instant cooling energy boost, **SPRAY THE SOLES OF THE FEET** with chilled cologne or rose geranium herbal water. For an even cooler sensation spray with chilled peppermint water.

133
SIGN OF THE TIMES

Beautiful nails are generally a sign of good health and good habits. Nails that are weak and brittle can be caused by dehydration, exposure to the elements, or cleaning chemicals. **Always protect the nails from harm by wearing gloves while cleaning.** Replace lost moisture by applying hand cream as often as skin and nails feel dry and taut.

Hand Facial

Apply a facial mask to back of hands once a month. Leave on for 10–15 minutes. Remove, rinse, and hydrate. Your hands will be smooth and wrinkles lessened. **Hands are the third place to reveal one's age.** *(First is the face, and second is the neck.)*

Play It Safe

DON'T USE YOUR FINGERNAILS AS TOOLS.

Instead, use a paper clip, screwdriver, or knife tip to pry something open.

Shape UP

Only shape the nails when they are dry.

If the nails are soft from the shower or bath, filing could cause splitting and breaking. Remember to file the nails in one direction. Toss metal files—they are too harsh. Opt for kinder, gentler instruments.

Give 'Em a Hand

A hand massage that is.

Using the thumb and index finger of your left hand, squeeze each finger on your right hand, one by one, and move the finger in small circles from your knuckles to your fingertips. Gently pull each finger, and then stretch the fingers backwards. Repeat on other hand. Using a hand cream with enriched moisturizers will help give your movements 'slip' and aid in massage efforts.

TiNY BUBBLES

To keep nail polish from bubbling up on nails, **DO NOT SHAKE THE POLISH.** Instead, turn the bottle upside down and roll gently between hands.

139

IN THE BUFF

Buffing the nail is the secret to building nail strength. By increasing the blood flow to the nail bed, the matrix of the nail is stimulated to grow. An added benefit is a smoother, shinier nail. Manicures last longer too.

Blister Buster

Petroleum Jelly lightly rubbed over the entire foot will eliminate friction and prevent blisters.

Also, hosiery is not as likely to get a run because of skin snagging.

COVER Up

For the softest hands and feet in town, once or twice a month, *slather on the* **richest hand cream** *you can find.* Slip on cotton socks and gloves for the night. Awake to supple, soft, and younger looking extremities.

Raise Your Hands

Make a commitment to beautiful nails.

Either schedule a weekly manicure appointment, or make a weekly date with yourself to do it at home. Our hands are always on display. Allow yours to look beautiful always.

Happy Feet

Schedule a pedicure once a month or pencil in a date to do it yourself.

Even in the dead of winter. When your toes are covered with socks and boots, you can secretly spice things up by painting your nails with 'rage red' or 'fantastic fuchsia'. Besides, when your toes peek out from under the bubbles in the bath, the bit of color will make you smile. Isn't that what life is all about?

SHAPE UP

MATCH YOUR PEDICURE POLISH TO YOUR TOENAIL SHAPE. Square toenails are most elegant with darker polish, on round toenails— classic reds or pinks look best.

145

De-puff

Relieve heat related puffiness in the fingers by soaking hands for **5** minutes in cold water mixed with sea salt.

The salt will pull the excess water from the hands.

Loosen Up

AVOID GETTING STIFF HANDS FROM REPETITIVE TASKS by opening and closing them under warm running water each time you wash your hands. As you dry them, feel each joint of each finger and gently massage them.

147

Green Thumb?

Rid your nails of dirt—especially working-in-the-garden dirt. Wet a nailbrush sprinkled with baking soda and gently scrub under running water. A better idea would be to use gardening gloves.

TOE TAPPING

To control stinky feet, try soaking the tootsies regularly in a footbath with a ½ cup of baking soda added to the water. Also, it's a great way to soothe tired, aching feet.

Smell gone and ache free—*sweet deal!*

NAiL iT

If your nails are prone to breaking, make sure that you get enough calcium, iron, and zinc in your diet to maintain strong, healthy nails. **Good foods to eat include raw vegetables, fresh fruit, and dairy products.** A nail, hair, and skin supplement is another excellent way to help from the inside out.

Made in the **SHADE**

Nails also need protection from the sun. Use a topcoat enriched with UVA and UVB filters. This will also help keep the nail polish from discoloring or looking dull.

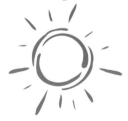

APPLY LIKE A *Pro*

To apply professional looking nail polish, paint one stripe down the middle of the nail from the base to the tip, then paint one brush stroke on each side. Make sure the coat is thin. Wait a few minutes, continue with second coat, and then end with a protective topcoat.

If the Shoe Fits. wear it.

But be careful of stylish, yet impractical footwear.
Bunions, calluses, and other foot maladies are
caused by shoes that don't fit properly. Sore
feet show all over the
face, body, and soul. It is
just not worth it!

Chapter 6

Bathing Rituals

"There must be quite a few things that a hot bath won't cure, but I don't know many of them."

Sylvia Plath

In the quiet calm of a bath, or in the stimulating zest of a shower, this daily ritual involves more than just getting clean. *It is about beautifying, grooming, connecting with your body, and refreshing your mind and soul.*

153

tub tips

Bathe without wrecking your hairdo. Just run a little cold water in the tub or shower first before turning on the hot. **This trick will prevent the hair-flattening steam clouds from ruining your 'Do.**

154

Deodorant soap will destroy your *perfume power*

These strong acting soaps are designed to fend off smells—of all kinds. *Using a lightly scented body wash or natural soap will keep your perfume fragrance lasting longer.* Although these items are scented also, the scent should not conflict or lessen the impact of your perfume.

155

GIVE ME TEN

Just 10 minutes in a relaxing tub of bubbles or aromatherapy oils can reduce stress and anxiety, and soothe tense and sore muscles. Even just replacing the rushed shower once a week will do wonders.

WASH AND GO

If your morning routine consists of jumping in the shower and jumping right out, **add some pizzazz** to your rush **hour with scented shower gels and luxurious body creams.** The extra minute it takes will add up to a more relaxed and focused morning commute.

M-M-M-GOOD

Create a rejuvenating spa with a sensuous milk bath. Mix one cup of powdered whole milk with one tablespoon of grapeseed oil and add to the running bath water. Just before you slide into the water add a few drops of your favorite essential oil. The milk contains lactic acid, which helps remove dead skin and grapeseed oil contains powerful antioxidants while the essential oils create a wonderful mood lifting fragrance. **CLEOPATRA HAD IT ALL FIGURED OUT!**

Too Hot To Handle

Shower or bath water that's **too hot will leave you feeling dehydrated and strip your skin of needed moisture.**

So, turn down the heat and preserve the skin.

Tea Party

Pick a teabag or two of your favorite herbal blend and tie the strings under the faucet so that the water will run through the bag. THE WATER WILL BE DELICIOUSLY SCENTED AND THE HERBAL BLEND WILL ADD SKIN-LOVING ANTIOXIDANTS TO THE BATH.

Take It Slow

Showers are mistakenly viewed as the stimulating side of bathing. But steamy, warm showers can be soothing and relaxing. **Linger longer and let the water massage your tense muscles.** Two extra minutes in the morning will set the calm factor for the day.

Outer Body Detox

Mix together ½ lb. of sea salt and 1 lb. of baking soda and add to a warm tub of water. Soak until the water is cool. This treatment is excellent for soothing itchy and dry skin. Plus it helps detoxify the skin by pulling out toxin waste from the pores.

OWN IT

Find one or two fragrances that you adore and make them your signature fragrances.

When people smell 'your signature' they will always think of you.

163
MAKE SCENT

Add a few drops of your signature fragrance to the rinse water of your fine washables such as hosiery and undergarments. You will take your special fragrance with you in a wonderfully understated way.

Luxury in a **BOX**

indulge in hard-milled body soaps.

Choose a scent each month and relish in the

wonderful aroma as you bathe.

SOAP

Smooth Operator

To keep ingrown hairs and 'orange peel' skin in check **gently loofah the bumpy skin or the areas that you shave while in the bath or shower.** Use small gentle circular motions. For an even better result, put an alpha hydroxy acid based product on the loofah before applying. This will help to remove dead skin. No pressure is necessary, but it should be done daily in order to beat the problem.

Indulging the 'scents'

Studies show that people who wear fragrance are found to have **improved moods** and **suffer less from anxiety and fatigue.** So pick yourself up and spritz a little on.

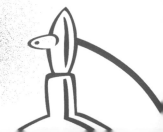

Running Hot And Cold

Taking a hot bath (100°F or 38°C) enhances the production of perspiration. The metabolism is stimulated so that increased amounts of the body's toxins are eliminated. Blood vessels and muscles relax in the cozy warmth so that you feel pleasantly relaxed. 15 to 20 minutes is perfect. A cold bath (54°F or 12.5°C) stimulates the metabolism, and quickens the cardiovascular and nervous systems. This bath is so stimulating that only 10 to 30 seconds is all that is needed to receive the full benefits.

Bottoms UP

To keep your backside as smooth as a baby's, exfoliate your bottom once a week.

This will stimulate blood circulation and make the skin more receptive to cellulite-firming treatments. Be sure to hydrate the area after treatment to ensure baby soft skin.

Elbow Room

The skin on the elbow is thicker and tougher than the rest of the arm, and is used constantly—leaning while writing, talking on the phone, or sitting in a chair. Too keep elbows soft and pretty, exfoliate while bathing. Then cut a grapefruit in half and place half under each elbow. Remain in this position for 15 minutes, letting them soak while you read your favorite book, (hopefully this one), or telephone a friend. The grapefruit will soften the skin while removing dark areas. *Grapefruit—it's not just for breakfast anymore.*

Baring It

Breast skin is very delicate and needs gentle care. Wash with lukewarm water and mild soap. If your skin seems drier than usual, use your facial moisturizing mask on the entire area twice a month. Rinse off in the shower. Breast skin will be softer, smoother, and more radiant.

Navel Fleet

The navel and stomach can be a beauty zone *(it does not have to be totally flat, it is very feminine to have a little roundness)*. The skin in this area is usually thicker and tougher but at the same time vulnerable to sagging or stretch marks. Cure? M&M. Moisturize and massage. Wash with a mild soap, and then apply moisturizer while massaging in circular motions until product is completely absorbed.

BACK UP *Plan*

The back is back. **Show it off, but be sure that it is as unblemished and s m o o t h as possible.**

Occasionally you may get unwanted pimples between your shoulders, where the oil glands are located. When this happens, cleanse the area with anti-bacterial soap, rinse, and then apply a drying lotion. Another idea—use a loofah daily in the shower to ward off any breakouts.

Body Rx

When your body skin needs extra moisture like after the bath or in the dead of winter, or very stressful situations, **give it a thorough beauty drink.** Wet yourself all over in the shower. Step out, apply moisturizer all over, go back in the shower, wash as usual, towel dry and then reapply a wonderfully hydrating cream and massage it in until the product is completely absorbed.

Masks Are Not
Just For Facials Anymore

Apply a good seaweed or mud mask on the back, legs, stomach, shoulders, or wherever you need an extra skin boost. It is a great remedy to skin problems such as dry skin, eczema, psoriasis, over active oil glands, and the like. Put a nice thick layer on and allow to dry. Hop in the shower and rinse off the treatment. Enjoy smoother and more toned skin.

Problem Solver Bath

For an achy, tired, nervous body—a wonderful remedy is to add 6 to 8 tablespoons of dry mustard to a hot bath and soak for about 20 minutes. Finish by rinsing in cooler water. The aches and pains are washed down the drain.

Now You're Cooking

Olive oil is an excellent skin moisturizer. This natural oil contains monounsaturated fat that easily absorbs into the skin leaving no residue. A little bit goes a long way. The skin is silky smooth, not greasy, and naturally refreshed.

177

Soak Your Head!

When a headache kicks in, **try soaking your feet in a basin of water mixed with one teaspoon of cayenne pepper for 10 minutes.** This treatment will draw the blood away from the head towards the feet, relaxing the body muscles and easing the headache. Say a-h-h-h-h.

MIND Detox

Relax your mind while enjoying your favorite bathing ritual, and take stock of your life. Reassess your lifestyle. Start by thinking of ways you can change it for the better, like cutting down on caffeine, adopting a healthier diet, or maybe joining a gym. Think about all of the good you can do for you.

LIKE Oil AND Water

They don't mix, no matter how you shake it. Capful after capful of bath oil poured in the tub will never make dry, flaky skin anymore hydrated. This is because oil and water simply do not mix and the only thing coated with the oil is the tub. New formulas of bath products are available that combine moisturizing ingredients dispensed in salts, foaming gels, or powders. You are left afterward with silky skin and the bath is not a slip and slide.

PUT IT – Don't Pour It

For those extremely dry skin areas, put on a thicker hydrating product. Creams don't 'pour' because they are thick with emollients and will moisturize deeper. Keep the pourable lotions for the normal skin areas, and for use in warmer weather.

181

Dish It Up

Plain oatmeal is a time-honored remedy that calms dryness and irritation by leaving a film on your skin that seals in water. Think of it as an invisible shield that fends off irritation and the urge to scratch. Easy to use, simply put one cup of uncooked oatmeal in an old stocking, or muslin bag, tie it and throw it into the tub as the water is filling. Soak for 10 to 15 minutes. DRY, ITCHY SKIN WILL BE A MEMORY.

WARD OFF Warts

Not a glamorous subject matter but a beauty buster for sure.

To avoid the condition altogether, be sure to cover your feet, especially around the gym and pool areas. Keep the feet dry. If your feet are moisture prone, use foot powder, and be sure to wear breathable shoes like leather or canvas. Always use a clean towel after bathing to reduce the likelihood of infection. Be careful when drying your feet and nails after cleansing, if there is a wart in the area and it is disturbed, it will suddenly become a colony of infection. At that point, see a doctor.

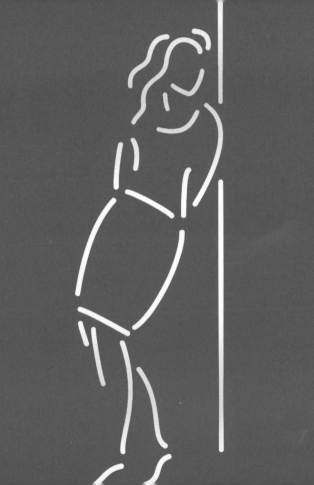

Chapter 7

Inside Out

"Everything you see, I owe to spaghetti."

Sophia Loren

Although genes have a great impact on how we look, how well we wear them is up to us. *Decide now to 'dress' yourself from the inside out to reflect the person you always knew you could be.*

Cut It Out

By reducing the caffeine, alcohol, refined sugar, flour, and junk foods in your diet, you will be increasing the benefits of vitamins and minerals metabolized in the body. The empty calorie foods deplete your body's stores of much needed nutrients.

PUMP IT UP

Exercise is more than just waist whittling. As the heart starts pumping, oxygen races around the body bringing with it nutrients to feed the skin cells. This action results in more collagen being produced, which improves the texture of the skin, and increases the blood flow to help keep the pores unclogged and free of grime. At the very least exercise gives the skin a wonderful healthy glow.

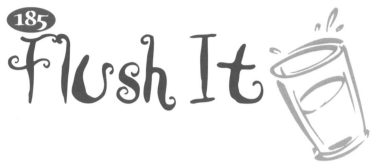

185 Flush It

Drinking 8 eight-ounce glasses of water each and every day will help flush the toxins away. For an added benefit, **drink it cold to help with weight control.** The body has to burn more calories when the water is cold.

Cough It Up

Quit smoking.

If you cannot quit for the health benefits alone, quit for your skin. Smoking is the second major cause of premature wrinkling (sun damage is the first). Nicotine constricts the small blood vessels and decreases the flow of oxygen and nutrients to your skin. Also, contorting the face by squinting the eyes and pulling the mouth when inhaling creates more lines on the face.

Just give it up!

SAY HEY BARTENDER

In excess, alcohol dehydrates the body and robs it of vitamins that keep skin both healthy and glowing. Make a promise to yourself that for every alcoholic beverage you consume, you will chase it with a glass of ice water with a splash of lemon or lime juice.

Mineral Reminder

In addition to building strong bones and teeth, calcium helps regulate healthy nerve and muscle functions.

A combination of calcium and magnesium acts as a mild relaxant and sleep promoter. Calcium, in addition to helping to combat osteoporosis, also helps to relieve premenstrual symptoms.

BYPASS the Buzz

Limit caffeine consumption.

Too much caffeine can make you fidgety and disturb your sleep. It restricts blood circulation making the skin's toxin-removing function less effective.

190 WORK IT

When working it, it is very important to exercise with a clean face to allow your pores to sweat out toxins. choose breathable cotton or cotton blends for clothing. Nylon and spandex against your skin trap moisture and toxins in. Shower after the workout to rid the skin of excreted toxins.

Process of **ELIMINATION**

To stay young and healthy, your digestion must function properly. Ridding the body of waste makes the difference between being sluggish and bloated or being vital and energized. Unless your body is efficiently eliminating daily, your metabolism will be slow, your stomach will protrude, and feeling 'out of sorts' will prevail.

Eat right, to rid right.

Move to LOSE

Regular exercise reduces the appetite, because it helps to control blood sugar levels and leads to a feeling of fullness.

Aerobic exercise reduces the appetite because it raises the body temperature.

Go for the Burn

Exercise in any form burns calories.

Regular exercise increases oxygen in the blood, improves heart and lung capacities, raises metabolism, promotes better digestion and enhances endurance and muscle tone. As an added bonus, exercise deters osteoporosis.

Cell-A-Brate

True beauty is never just skin deep.

Beauty comes from deep inside the soul and

radiates through each cell. The inside of our cells

definitely shows on the outside.

Numbers Game

'Ideal weight' is about as truthful as 'one size fits all.'

Beauty does not count numbers, it counts confidence in whatever the scale says. A healthy, toned body can be several scale measures away from the so-called 'ideal' and still be just the right size for you. *Trust your instincts.*

Get the Juice

Raw fruits and vegetables, especially freshly squeezed juices, increase the level of enzymes in the body. By incorporating fresh juice into your daily diet, **you will be drinking your way to better** health and becoming **younger to boot!**

Sigh of Relief

For a natural, yet effective breath freshener, mix one-half teaspoon of baking soda in a cup of water and rinse the mouth. The baking soda will neutralize all odors, onion, garlic, and even the notorious morning breath! Plus it will leave you with a fresh taste as opposed to an alcohol taste.

THE 'Cat Walk'

Don't compare yourself to the seemingly 'flawless' supermodels you see in the magazines. Did you know that it usually takes 5–10 rolls of film to get that 'natural' cover shot? Remember that computers are the best 'beautifiers'—a bit off there, a color change here, add a little cleavage, take away a little waist; and on and on. **EVEN THE WICKED WITCH OF OZ COULD BE BEAUTIFUL WITH ENOUGH GAUZE OVER THE LENS!**

LAST ON, First off

The last place you put on weight will be the first place that you lose it. That stubborn, 'always-bothered-you' part (or parts) of your body will take a while to lose. But take heart, with a sensible eating and a thorough exercising plan you will lose fat and get to all those 'bothersome' areas.

Funny Face

Find something to laugh at—a really 'hold your side and laugh about it' something everyday. Not only is it great for your soul, but it helps with weight loss, too! The calories burned are the equivalent of climbing two flights of stairs.

Laugh it off!

201

Sleep on It

Taking Evening Primrose oil and vitamin E capsules before retiring allows the body to absorb these powerful anti-agers into the system during it's most restorative time of rest.

Ginseng to Me

Ginseng is an excellent supplement to improve your energy levels and mental alertness. Reports show that it has immune strengthening benefits and helps to lower cholesterol levels. It is also used in beauty and health products to 'wake' up the skin.

Tag-A-Long

For best absorption, take vitamins and supplements with meals. The stomach juices are more active when digesting food, allowing the nutrients to enter the system more quickly.

Tick-Tock-Not!

Ticking clocks will not do if you are really trying to get some beauty sleep. The constant tick-tock will not soothe you to sleep but rather cause you to count each and every second. Opt instead for a silent digital clock. And turn the clock face away so that you are not constantly checking it during the night. Don't worry, it will wake you when the right time comes.

205

Dole it Out

If you suffer from premenstrual syndrome (PMS) INCLUDE JUICE MADE FROM PINEAPPLE IN YOUR DIET. Pineapples contain an enzyme called bromelain. It has a soothing, relaxing effect on the body's muscle tissue which helps to ease menstrual cramping.

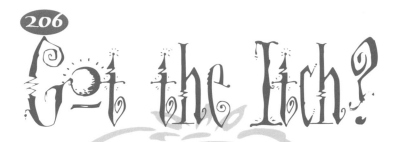

Got the Itch?

Eating more foods that are rich in bioflavonoids such as sweet pepper, tomatoes, parsley, and cabbage **will help reduce surface inflammation.** Eating foods containing zinc, such as carrots, garlic, and ginger, and essential fatty acids such as fish, nuts, and seeds will lessen eczema symptoms.

Banish **THE BLOAT**

Increasing your intake of potassium-rich foods such as bananas, prunes, raisins, figs, seaweed, broccoli, spinach, fish, green vegetables, celery, and apples **will help reduce body fluid retention.** Juices made from watermelon, cucumber, and grapes will also help to **rid the system of excess water.**

Breathe Deep, *Sleep Tight*

Eating pineapple will help reduce sinus congestion, and assist with sleeping problems.

It is also used as an anti-inflammatory treatment for arthritis, and it aids in reducing fluid retention.

So Mad that You Could Chew Nails?

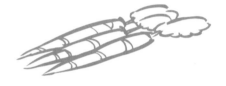

Opt instead for raw vegetables. **Munching on crunchy, good-for-you foods helps reduce frustration and tension.**

Carrots (and other vegetables) can help you cope!

Hot Flashes are not that Hot

If you suffer from sudden feelings of overheating due to a rush of hormones or being in a overheated room, have a spot of tea. Hot tea like peppermint tea will have an instant cooling effect on the system, believe it or not. *Next time a woman's* **'power surge'** *hits, it's teatime.*

211

Take an Air Bath

Enjoy the total freedom of walking around your home in your birthday suit. Of course, remember to adjust the blinds. Turn on some relaxing music and just feel the freedom. You will feel like a kid again.

HIP TO BE SQUARE

Consuming 3 square meals a day is vital if you want to kick-start your metabolism and keep it humming all day long. By eating every 3 to 5 hours, you will avoid the mid-morning energy slump and the afternoon goodie cravings.

Food's Bad Boys

Don't be fooled by diet foods. Be it 'lite' mayonnaise or 'diet' pudding, all the rich, quality foods that we love come in lighter, fat-free, no sugar added versions. These foods may be less fattening, but since the flavor is not quite the same, we have a tendency to eat more, thus defeating the purpose. Instead enjoy the real thing in moderation. You will be more satisfied and you'll avoid those mystery chemicals found in 'fake' food.

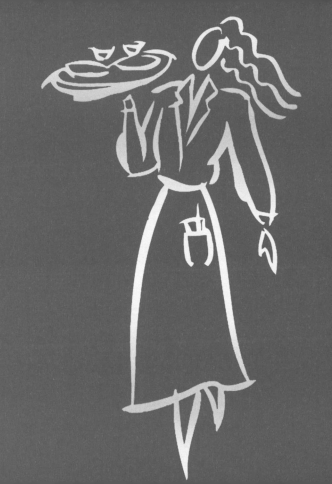

Chapter 8

Beauty Bytes

"One cannot think well, love well, sleep well, if one has not dined well."
Virginia Woolf

eauty comes from deep within. A proper eating regime of healthy, nutritious foods will show in all ways—in all places. From the top of your head, to the bottom of your feet, *the body is a living example of what you eat.*

Beans, Beans,
THE MAGICAL FOOD

The more you eat them, the better your mood. Beans are high in the B vitamins, known to be mood stabilizers. They are also high in complex carbohydrates, magnesium, iron, zinc, and fiber. A cup a day is all you need.

Peel It

High in natural sugar, bananas are wonderful, self-contained packages of quick, healthy energy. A good source of potassium and magnesium, as well as other essential minerals and vitamins plus soluble and insoluble fibers, bananas are just plain 'appealing.' Add a few of these energy boosters to your diet weekly.

An Apple A Day

Apples are tasty, easy to carry and quench the desire for something sweet.

They're rich in both soluble and insoluble fiber, potassium, and trace minerals. Keep the Doctor away? It sure could not hurt.

C–Me

Oranges are chock full of skin healthy, cold-fighting vitamin C, and soluble and insoluble fibers, anti-aging bioflavonoids, folic acid, and potassium. A great way to start the morning.

SEE THE GREEN

Broccoli is a nutritional wonder. Just a few servings weekly will deliver plenty of vitamin C, some A and B complex, and other minerals especially calcium and magnesium. Plus broccoli is famous for it's fiber—enjoy!

Sesame Street

Sesame seeds, although tiny, store a lot of absorbable calcium and magnesium. They are also high in fiber and trace minerals. Just 2 tablespoons sprinkled over your salad or vegetables every day will make a major impact on your daily mineral intake.

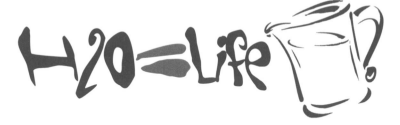

Water is a wondrous thing.

It keeps you feeling full, hydrates your skin, keeps your organs humming, and rids the body of toxins effectively. Drink at least 8 glasses daily, and more if your level of activity, warrants it.

Shell It Out

Shellfish, (shrimp, clams, scallops, lobster, crab, conch, crayfish, oysters, prawns, or snails) is a wonderful, low calorie, and nutritionally sound choice when adding protein to your program. All are high in the beauty nutrients such as the B vitamins, iron, iodine, zinc, and copper. Opt for one of these, once or twice a week.

KING FISH

Salmon is known as the king of omega-3 fats which are known for their ability to help lessen the symptoms of PMS as well as other maladies. Plus omega-3 fats are excellent skin nutrients. CROWN YOURSELF ONCE A WEEK.

whole world

Eat a proper, balanced diet with as many whole, unrefined foods as possible.

Reducing the amount of refined, over-processed, sugary foods will not only clean up your insides, but also help combat weight gain and water retention.

SLEEK PHYSIQUE

Avoid salty foods at all costs.

Salt causes your body to retain water, which, of course, makes the skin look puffy and bloated. Retained water is a major influence on the appearance of the dreaded cellulite. Opt for salt-free seasonings instead.

225

Detox Daily

Start the day with a quick and effective body detox drink. Squeeze the juice of ½ lemon or lime into a mug. Add hot water and drink slowly. This daily ritual will help flush out all the impurities that your body has managed to pick up overnight and prepare your skin for a new day.

SPICE IT UP

Spicy foods such as salsa, mustard, chili, and peppers can raise the body's metabolic rate allowing it to burn more calories. In fact, up to 50% more calories are burned when the food is on the hot and spicy side. Say okay to Ole!

GO FOR BLUE

Blueberries are excellent collagen promoters. Skin collagen helps reduce wrinkling. So just maybe ½ cup of blueberries a few times a week could keep the plastic surgeon away!

SUNNY SIDE UP

Breakfast eaters are typically more energetic and in turn can perform work tasks more efficiently. Plus studies show that breakfast eaters think more creatively. So start thinking about what you want for breakfast!

DON'T SKIP IT

Skipping breakfast could make you fatter!

Breakfast eaters are slimmer than non-breakfast eaters. By starting your day in a healthy way, the temptation to grab a doughnut or some other nutritionally void, sweet and gooey mid-morning snack is diminished.

FOOD OF THE ANGELS

Chocolate, a little indulgence that is good for you, contains magnesium, antioxidants, and heart-healthy compounds. Besides, splurging is good for you—period.

Souper

Instead of the grab-and-go lunch, savor a bowl of soup. Soup sipping encourages slower, relaxed meals. Plus as an extra bonus, people who begin their meal with soup consume fewer calories. Now that is souper douper!

232

INNOVATE DON'T Vegetate

Try a new vegetable.

Why not try broccoli rabe, or celery root, or

better yet, add lots of new veggies to a soup.

They're colorful in your bowl and good for you!

Eat something new this week.

233

Table For One?

You can still enjoy the bounty of fresh, roadside produce stops. Feel the fruit, smell the freshness of the vegetables, then buy a basket of each. Ask for extra bags and share the bounty with neighbors and friends. You will eat right and make new friends.

Arouse the Taste Buds

Make a Mediterranean inspired salad. Add pears, provolone cheese, arugula, fresh basil, tomatoes, and olives. Drizzle champagne vinaigrette on top. **Enjoy!**

Out with the Old, In with the New

For the most aromatic and delicious dishes, **invest in new spices.** Throw out all that are cakey, and over a year old. The delightful wake-up-the-palate-feeling is worth the effort. Plus when you cook, always make it your best effort—use only fresh and new produce. Would you expect any less if you were eating out?

Salt of the Earth

Too much sodium causes bloating, fluid retention, to say nothing about the health problems caused by excess salt. To help you kick the added salt trap, try removing the saltshaker from the table, or at least switch the saltshaker top with that of the pepper (the salt usually has 5 holes while the pepper has only 2 or 3). Try herbal spice blends that jazz up the food without adding the bloat!

237

Don't DILUTE

Drinking water, tea, and the like with meals dilutes the nutrients from the food by flushing the food too quickly through the system. By all means drink your daily water, **but skip it at meal times for the best absorption of body helping food nutrients.**

Tootsie Roll® Control

What if you absolutely, positively, must have a sweet treat or you will die? **A TOOTSIE ROLL POP® IS A GOOD AND SWEET TREAT.** With only 60 calories, it is a long lasting sweet satisfaction that few other foods can match. So when your sweet tooth is aching for a treat, lick (don't chomp) a Tootsie Roll Pop® in your favorite flavor.

Egg it On

Eggs are good for you. Eating eggs a couple of times a week will offer an excellent source of protein to your diet while adding only 70 calories each. A delicious vegetable loaded omelet with sliced tomatoes makes a great meal—at any time.

Lettuce See

The darker the color of lettuce, or any green vegetable for that matter, the more vitamins and minerals they contain. Romaine, red leaf, green leaf, and butter head lettuces also contain more iron than that wimpy iceberg lettuce. So toss the iceberg—out the door. Stick to the healthy kinds.

241

Hey Sugar!

Stevia, a South American herb, is calorie free and has the sweetening power of **200** times that of sugar. Healthfood stores are the easiest place to find it. Use this natural, non-chemical alternative to the little pink and blue packs—which contain all kinds of unpronounceable ingredients. Ugh!

First Class —Even in Economy

When flying, request a special meal such as low fat or vegetarian.

You will get colorful, appetizing food with fruit and vegetables rather than over cooked and over greased mystery meat. Plus they serve the special meals first, so you'll feel first class and avoid some calories!

CAN IT!

Put canned meats, soups, or gravies that contain fat in the refrigerator. **When you open them, the fat will be right on top.** Simply take a spoon and remove the fat before preparing and avoid the extra calories without sacrificing the flavor.

244

Prime **THE PUMP**

After exercising for 20 minutes or more, eat a high-quality nutrient food within 30 minutes of finishing your workout. Your tired muscles will be depleted of vital nutrients and are primed to soak up energy. Plus the nutrients will be used to replenish the hardworking muscle cells and are less likely to convert to fat cells.

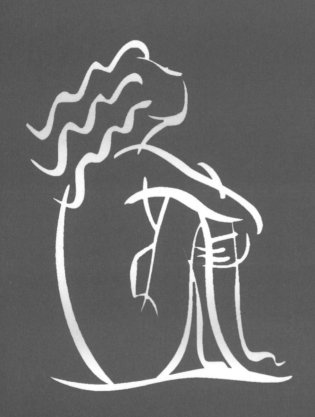

Chapter 9

In The Details

"If a woman knows she's pretty, it's not because some other woman told her so."   Anonymous

Beauty is more than lotions, potions, powders, and creams. Although these items are essential to create and maintain beauty—*it's the details that make the difference.* The behind-the-scene tips on grooming and lifestyle enhancements are the little extra touches that allow beauty to emerge as an art form.

H2-O My!

Water is the number one beauty treatment—period.

You cannot create beauty without beginning with a clean, clear canvas. If you are not drinking at least eight to ten glasses daily, you are depriving yourself of the best beauty secret on earth.

246

LAY ME DOWN

Invest in *silk or satin* pillowcases. They are more slippery than cotton, so your skin is less likely to be squished into wrinkle-inducing folds.

247

Take Control

The payoffs for indulging in beauty treatments are much more than skin deep. Spa experts now realize that if you consciously include some extra me-time into your schedule, you start to feel more powerful and more in control of your life. **Make an appointment with your favorite spa for a facial, manicure or massage—or all three,** and enjoy the benefits.

Every Breath You Take

Good skin comes with every breath you take, if you take it right. The skin is gasping for oxygen. Stomach breathing brings much needed, life-affirming oxygen to each skin cell. As you take a deep breath, place one hand on your stomach and the other on your chest. Check to see which hand is moving. If it is the hand on your stomach, congratulations you are giving your cells what they need. If the hand on your stomach is stationary and the hand on your chest is moving, take action—start breathing more deeply from your stomach area by pushing the stomach way out when inhaling and collapsing it when exhaling. Breathe deep and often.

SLEEPING BEAUTY

While you are sleeping, a special skin-growth hormone is released to boost the production of collagen and keratin (the proteins that make up your skin cells) and encourage cell turnover. Lose sleep and your skin will reflect it by being dull and dry with dark circles around your eyes. Try to get your rest, remember *it is not called BEAUTY sleep for nothing.*

FAKE IT, Don't Bake It

You cannot afford a suntan. The damage caused

by exposure to the sun is responsible for 80% of

all skin damage. Play it safe and

fake it with a self-tanner— only

you will know the difference.

251
SLEEP SANS *Makeup*

Going to bed with makeup on takes 10 days off the life of the face. The tossing and turning grinds the makeup into the pores and causes clogs and grime to go deeper. The eyelashes also take a beating by being squished with dried, cakey mascara, causing them to break off. Just two minutes is all it takes to preserve your skin.

Light Up Your Life

Wearing light colored clothing reflects light up and onto the face. The skin will look more alive and have a beautiful *glow*.

253

No Brow **Ow!**

Tweeze eyebrows when the skin is less sensitive. Sensitive times include first thing in the morning, because the skin tends to be puffy; after experiencing the outdoor cold or hot temperatures, as the skin will be trying to compensate for weather conditions; and it is best to avoid brow shaping while having your monthly cycle when the skin nerve endings are apt to be the most sensitive. *The best time is right after a shower because the pores are open and the hair easier to remove.*

Over Pluck – YOU'RE STUCK!

Be careful not to over tweeze the brows. BROW HAIR IS THE MOST UNPREDICTABLE HAIR ON THE BODY.

It might not grow back. Best advice, have them done professionally then 'clean up' the re-growth between visits.

255

Never Economize On The Luxuries

When you decide to splurge and truly pamper yourself, loosen up the purse strings. Luxuries are meant to be enjoyed without guilt and with a 'priceless' concern.

Wake Up Call

Start the day off with a total body glow.
First thing in the morning bend over at the waist as far as you can, hold your ankles and count to 30. Rise up slowly. Your circulation is boosted, and blood flows through the skin allowing for better skin cell turnover.

257

Bounce® it Out!

if skin is naturally sensitive, avoid fabric softener or dryer sheets when laundering towels, washcloths, sheets or pillowcases. The static reducing ingredient is a known skin-sensitizing agent. Also some of the products contain pore-clogging ingredients that can cause breakouts.

Looking Glass

A **3X** or **5X** magnifying mirror is a gal's best friend. You can get a heads up on sunspots, wrinkles and especially those pesky facial hairs (or as they are fondly called 'witch hairs') that occur seemingly overnight. Also it's always a good idea to give yourself the once over in the tell-all mirror everyday before leaving the house.

DON'T GET STUCK

Just because it 'worked' for you at 25 doesn't mean that it will work at 35 and beyond. Update your look—hair, makeup, and clothes need to keep up with the times. **A dated look is a dead look.**

YUK IT UP!

A good laugh is the **'tranquilizer with no side effects.'** Laughing reduces stress hormone levels, lowers blood pressure, and relieves muscle tension. Plus by increasing blood circulation, your skin is fed with life affirming oxygen.

Pretty Is As Pretty Does

As corny as it seems, feel pretty and that is what the world will see. Feel ugly and it will show all over your entire persona. *Try to look as good as you can each day and let your confidence show.*

Looking GOOD

There is no shame in wanting to look and feel your best. Appearance still matters. Caring for yourself physically inside and out will help you feel good emotionally. **True beauty includes exercise, proper nutrition, and self-acceptance.** Flaunt it.

Once Over

A couple of times during your day set aside **5 minutes** to give yourself the once over. Check your makeup, hair, clothing, and posture. Even if you begin the day perfect, a touch up is warranted to keep the perfect look going. Afterwards take a few deep breaths to instantly refresh your mind and you are all set.

Live In BEAUTY

Find a space that you can dedicate to beauty. Make it a special place just for you to enjoy your beauty rituals. Make a place that has everything at your fingertips to allow you to 'get it together' with ease. Not only will you feel more organized, but more confident as well. *The professionals keep everything in its place, and you should too.*

FIRST IMPRESSIONS LAST

Within 10 seconds of meeting someone, they form up to 11 opinions about you.

Everything from your financial status to your character is judged. What impressions do you want to leave them with?

Face Off

Be careful where you put your face.

Telephone receivers, both ear and mouthpiece, continually rub against the skin piling on bacteria, old makeup, and grime. Clean the phone regularly. Also make it a habit to keep your hands off your face. Remind yourself not to prop. Hands pick up all kinds of grime. Yuk!

I See

EYEGLASSES AND SUNGLASSES CAN CAUSE BUMPS, CYSTS, AND/OR BLACKHEADS UNDER THE FRAMES.

Clean the frames often with a mild detergent and rinse. If problems persist, check to make sure that your eye cream is oil-free.

And I Quote:

"There is no such thing as an ugly woman, only a lazy one."

Helena Rubenstein and I agree.

There is no reason not to make yourself look as good as you can. A good beauty routine should take you no more than 15 minutes from cleaning the skin to complete makeup application. Throw in a shower, and hair styling and you have 45 minutes tops! Life is not a dress rehearsal, what are you saving it for?

269

IN THE CLOSET

if it needs cleaning, clean it.

if it needs tossing, toss it.

if it needs repairing, do it now.

Nothing can spread stress faster than 5 minutes

to dress and nothing to wear!

Strike A Pose

Practice posing for photographs in front of a mirror. Look at your smile, do your eyes twinkle? Do you look natural? If you practice now, you will look perfectly natural for those candid shots in which you usually had your mouth open or all of your fillings were showing. Say cheese!

271

Internal Clock

The body works in rhythms. Sleeping late on weekends could disturb your body clock for the upcoming week. However, going to bed a little earlier does not seem to have that effect. So try to catch the extra

Z-Z-Z-Z-Zs

the night before to keep your clock ticking on time.

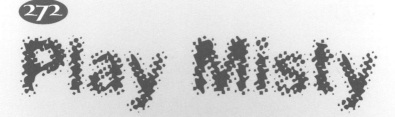

Play Misty

For the most hydrated winter skin, invest in a room (or even a whole house) humidifier. Not only is it good for dry, itchy, flaky skin but your wood furnishings, upholstery, and plants will also benefit. Plus you will breathe easier with moist air surrounding you.

273

FILTERING IN

Changing the air and humidifier filters does not sound like a beauty tool, but it is. *Cleaning filters often keeps dust, dirt, pollen and the like away from the skin, the eyes and the breathing passages.*

Check yours now!

SHED YOUR SKIN

Washcloths and towels need to be changed often. When towels dry the body, the terry cloth naturally exfoliates the skin. When the towel is used repeatedly, the old exfoliated skin cells will cling to the damp body causing itchy skin. Change washcloths morning and night. In the morning, the cloth removes spent out toxins from sleeping, in the evening the cloth removes the makeup and dirt from the day. For the freshest skin—use fresh linens.

MOUNTAIN HIGH

Bring along the sunscreen and hat.

Just because your summer holiday plans are not centered around the beach, doesn't mean that you are sun safe. In fact, higher elevations mean less atmosphere to screen the sun's rays—causing the skin to burn faster—double that burn rate if your vacation plans include a winter wonderland of skiing. Take it along and slather it on.

Chapter 10

The Good Life

"Too much of a good thing is wonderful." Mae West

Scheduling in private time on a daily basis is what the good life is all about. *The coveted 'alone-time' is a great way to rediscover your wonderful uniqueness.*

276

Sit Right Down

Instead of telephoning or e-mailing a friend, *write a good old-fashioned letter.* Use pretty stationery or note cards, a fancy pen and write in longhand. Enclose a photograph or two of a place that you have recently traveled to, or a picture of you and your pen pal. It is so much fun to retrieve a letter from the mailbox written especially to you.

Nature Calls

Experience nature by getting out and walking for just 20 minutes.

Focus on the scenery, the sounds of nature, and the rhythm of your breathing. Feel your muscles move you forward, as you re-count all of the things for which you are grateful.

278

Keep It Fresh

Keep fresh flowers in your home. It is an easy way to add beauty and bring the refreshing scents of nature inside all year long. Flowers lift the spirit. For about the same amount as a trip to the gourmet coffee house you can give yourself an inexpensive gift that will last all week.

Tea Anyone?

As an every afternoon treat do as the English do and have a 'spot' of tea. Green tea is full of healthy antioxidants. Steep in a porcelain teapot and serve in a dainty china cup and saucer; add lemon and even a fruit scone if you would like. Enjoy this age-old ritual.

280

Right Away

Sign up for a creative workshop.

Develop your right brain by attending an art, music or writing class. If you cannot find a class, host a gathering of like-minded friends to discuss the arts, or maybe even start a book club.

TALENT SHOW

Regardless of what your talent is, it cannot be developed without a clear mind. Your talent is only as good as your health; **so with good health you have the time and energy to develop your talent to the fullest.**

WHAT CHA' DOING?

At this very moment, you are using your free time to read this book. But how do you use the rest of your free time? And why do you spend your free time the way that you do?

PLUG IN DAILY

To nourish your inner self during the day, pick a 5-minute slot of time and really concentrate on your breathing. Relax each body part one at a time and truly feel the sensation. Concentrate on the areas of your body where you store tension. **Just 5 minutes every day of concentrated deep breathing and focusing on each and every part of yourself will increase endurance and reduce stress.**

Prepare For STRESS

The unfortunate news is that if you are not stressed now, you probably will be soon. When you are frazzled, your ability to handle stress is diminished. So plan ahead. Make a list of 10 things that make you feel happy and alive. Maybe it is taking a walk, immersing in a bubble bath, calling a really good friend and just laughing about whatever it is—anything that makes you feel better and your life easier. When you are overburdened, take out the list. Just pick one thing and do it!

285

Speed Limit

Slow down and *relax*.

Racing around at breakneck speed is surely not the way to enjoy life. Pace yourself and your 'things to do list.' Be sure to factor in some creative thinking time.

Accentuate The Positives

Keep a positive attitude.

Thinking negatively not only affects your mood, and your performance, it shows on your face and in your health in general. Plus 'stinking thinking' affects the people around you, and no one wants to be around a downer—even for a minute.

287

Keep It Simple

Remember it is the simple things that bring the greatest joys. **Count your blessings not your money.** Smile more and wrinkle less. By laughing you will exercise your facial muscles and keep them toned. Remember, they call them frown lines for a reason.

Dear Diary

Keep a daily journal beside your night table.
Each night take a moment and write down your
reflections of the day. It is an excellent way to let
go, unwind and allow the day to fade away. As you
end the evening journaling, jot down two things
that you like about yourself and why.

Glam It Up

Make your bedroom your haven.
Surround yourself with colorful pillows to lounge on while reading or writing. Keep photos of great experiences around you to remember how much fun life is. Have pretty sheets to sleep on and wear something that makes you feel special. Spray the sheets with lavender to relax, and replace your night table light bulb with a pink tinted one. You will like the way your skin looks.

Unplugged

Turn off the Palm Pilot,® computer, answering machine, fax, beeper, cell phone and make believe that you have been cast away on a tropical island. **See if you can be technology free for one day.** You will find that messages in a bottle work just as well.

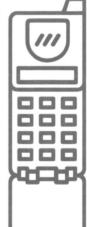

SEEING GREEN

Believe it or not, houseplants are beauty aids. They help purify the air and counteract allergies—even helping to eliminate headaches! Surround your home with greenery for beauty in decorating and for the skin! Don't forget to water!

HIDDEN LUXURY

Paint the inside of your closet with your favorite color. Add a beautiful border of fabric along the top. Add colorful storage bins. Paste photos of styles you admire on the inside door. You will smile every time you open the door and will enjoy your daily dressing ritual a whole lot more.

OUTSIDE IN

Bring a bit of the outdoors inside.

Put wooden trays or zinc buckets of green grass around your living spaces. You can't help but run your fingers (or toes) through it when you pass by. Seeing growing, living things is good for your health and refreshes your soul.

THE GETAWAY

Be ready for an escape weekend. Always keep a waterproof toilette bag packed with travel sizes of all of your can't live without products. That way, you'll be ready to seize the moment – in a moment's notice!

Be Selfish

At least once a day do something

that is just for you. Don't feel guilty—

remember it is your life—you deserve it!

296

Be Generous

At least twice a day do something

for someone who needs help.

You'll feel extra good if you do it anonymously.

Silence Is Golden

Take a mental vacation by not talking for a

minimum of two hours. Think, read, write, or

reflect on your blessings instead. YOU WON'T

MISS THE CHATTER — TRUST ME.

Take A Week off

Turn off the TV for a week.

Listen to music, or read instead. It will be like a mini-mental sabbatical. When (or if) you resume watching TV you will find that you did not miss much, the same people are in the news, and the shows are still focusing on the same old topics.

A Bit Of Good Humor

BE IN A GOOD MOOD. IT IS CONTAGIOUS.

Smile and say hello to everyone you meet. Give a sincere compliment to three people every day. Your facial muscles will relax, you will put some pep in your step, and your compliment will make someone's day. Think about how you feel when you get one. Go out and give three a day!

Time Out

Give yourself permission to take naps once in a while.

There is nothing more delicious than an after Sunday brunch nap. Cover yourself with a silk throw and drift off for an hour or so. Awake refreshed and wonderfully relaxed.

301

Keep In Touch

Buy vintage postcards and send them to friends you would normally e-mail or phone. There is something about a personally written note, on a lovely postcard, that says classic!

Vacation Without Leaving Town

If you can't get away for a vacation, at least

book a weekend at a luxury hotel with a spa.

Rent a sporty car to get you to your destination.

You will feel like you're on the sunny Riviera!

303

SAY O-M-M-M-M-M-M

MEDITATING FOR 5 MINUTES A DAY
IS A GREAT WAY TO BOOST YOUR
SELF-ESTEEM AND SELF-CONFIDENCE.

Five minutes a day every day.
Surely you can find the
time. You just spent a
minute or two reading
this message!

304

Calming Light

Drop a tiny bit of oil of lavender on a light bulb, or ceramic bulb ring. The heat of the bulb diffuses the uplifting and relaxing scent of lavender throughout the entire room.

Candlelight

Besides providing a wonderful glow, scented candles create a mood in the home that is relaxing, soothing, and stress-easing. Keep several throughout your home and enjoy them daily—not just when company comes.

Here's Mud In Your Eye

Not on the carpet.

If you are going to use at-home, spa mud or herbal wrap treatments invest in a small plastic stool. Put it in the shower or bathtub to provide a place to sit while the treatment works. Bring a book and relax while the products work. Afterward shower off the treatment and the stool. All clean—without the mess!

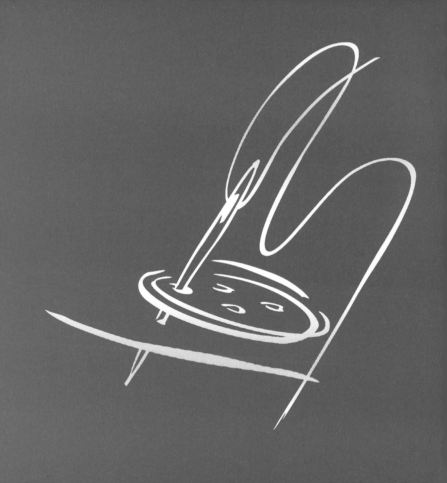

Chapter 11

Quick Fix Remedies

"The beautiful is not always expensive, and the expensive is not always beautiful." Unknown

Sometimes we are faced with an uh-o beauty crisis for which a solution is needed ASAP. Other times, knowing what to do before it happens is of great help. *In both situations, a smart, quick fix remedy is worth its weight in gold.*

DE-PUFFERY

For swollen eyelids, dip cotton balls or cosmetic squares into cold whole milk or cream. Lie down, and apply soaked cotton to your eyelids. Leave on for 5 to 10 minutes. The high fat content of either liquid provides a moisturizing treatment for the delicate, thin skin around the eyes.

ODORS OUT

To rid the hands and fingers of onion, garlic, and yes, even tobacco odors rub them with a slice of lemon or lime and rinse with water. Apple cider vinegar also works. Dry hands and apply hand cream, odors are vanished, and hands are kissable once again.

Eye Believe

Treat yourself to an aromatic herbal eye pillow.

Lie down, close your eyes, and drape the sooth-

ing, calming herb scented pillow gently over your

eyes. Just 10 minutes will do you a world of good.

You will emerge anew. Now doesn't that feel better?

310
GET THE RED OUT

To lessen the redness of a blemish, apply a small amount of an eye drop product designed for tired eyes to the blemish. The active ingredient will help remove the redness and calm things down.

A Little Dab Will Do You

For a quick remedy for a pimple, put

a pea-sized dollop of toothpaste on

the bump before going to bed.

Overnight the blemish will dry up and almost vanish.

Take The Cure

Ease a hangover by soaking in a tub of hot water scented with fennel, juniper and rosemary oils. Drink plenty of water with squeezed lemons, limes, or oranges in it. Put a lavender scented cloth over your eyes and try to remember that this will pass. But also try to remember to stop a couple of drinks earlier next time.

One-Minute Refresher

When your eyes are just too tired to focus on anything, try this little trick. Close your eyes and cup the palms of your hands over each eye for at least one minute. The tiny reprieve in the dark will lessen strain and instantly refresh the eyes.

Shake It

If your loose powder seems to go everywhere but on your face, trade the box for a shaker—a salt shaker. Put the powder in a clean and dry salt-shaker then you simply shake some out into your hand, swish around your powder brush and apply. **Perfect application—and no messy clothes or countertops!**

315

DON'T STOP CHANGING

You owe it to yourself to keep up with the times and the styles. If not, you will end up looking out of date, out of style, and like a caricature of yourself or like the photos of yourself you would rather not pull out in public. **The quickest beauty fix is to keep up with what's what!**

SMOOTH OPERATOR

To make your leg shaving last longer, before shaving, lightly rub a loofah or washcloth over the entire area. This will help shed the dead skin and any skin oils, allowing for a closer, longer lasting shave. Be sure to moisturize the skin afterwards for the ultimate in silky smooth skin.

317
Midnight Express

The body does most of its repair work on the skin between the hours of 1AM and 4AM. Don't miss the train! Be sure to 'pack' on the proper skin care products before retiring to make the most difference in your skin. All aboard!

Ears Looking At You

Ears are one of the most sensual beauty zones.

For an instant beauty lift, expose them often. Try the hair behind one or both ears. Wear statement earrings to bring more attention to this 'ear-resist-able' area.

319

Marks The Spot

For a quick overview of whether your skin is sensitive, with your clean thumbnail, gently make a X between your brows. If the redness remains for a while, your skin is sensitive in addition to your usual skin type (i.e. normal/ sensitive, oily/sensitive, etc).

WHEN A RE-DO WON'T DO

Sometimes you have to wash, tone, and hydrate during the middle of the day due to excess oiliness, or maybe you just need to pretend to start your day over again. Keep sample or trial sizes of your facial regime as well as cosmetics you'll need for a quick makeover—like wet/dry foundation which will also act as a powder, a blush that can double as eye shadow, mascara, and lipstick. Keep in a small travel bag with a mirror. Now suddenly you are a new you—and it's only lunchtime!

Smitten With Mittens

For an alternative to once again blow drying your hair, try a new approach. Terry cloth mittens, usually found in the travel department or a drug store are perfect for drying hair gently. Go over the hair several times with the mittens, and then take areas of hair between the mittens. Perfect summer vacation hair-tousled yet chic.

322
Sharpen Up

To sharpen blunt tweezers, gently run extra fine sandpaper over the inner tips. Rinse

and dry. Now you can get that 'wild hair' with ease.

SHOPPED 'TIL YOU DROPPED?

Revive tired, aching feet by rubbing the soles with a washcloth dipped in apple cider vinegar for 3 minutes on each foot. Massage feet and toes with the cloth soaked mixture and then let the feet air-dry. Happy feet have now returned.

EEK STREAKS!

When your self-tanner leaves you with streaks of uneven color, smooth whitening toothpaste onto streak marks.

Leave on several minutes to lighten discoloration.

Rinse off with warm water. Telltale landing strip lines will have vanished.

325

Sight For Sore Eyes

If, after being exposed to extremely harsh weather—hot or cold, your eyes look like road maps of red lines, or they ache to beat the band, try applying cold compresses of chamomile tea bags to the eyelids for 5 minutes. *Do yourself a favor and fix yourself a cup of the relaxing tea, saving the bags for the eyes.* Prop up your feet, put the bags on your eyes, and think about how much better you feel already.

Make Scents

Clean a perfume atomizer by rinsing it with vodka, **then with water** before filling it with a new scent.

The vodka neutralizes the previous aroma allowing for the new fragrance to fully blossom.

MORE *For* Less

You will get more mileage from your lipstick if you apply it with a lip brush. It is estimated that by using a lip brush you will get an additional twenty or more applications. Plus, by using a lipstick brush, you can put it precisely where you want it. *And let's face it, using a lip brush is just downright more glamorous.*

Tight Squeeze

Did you know that between the ages of 20 and 50 your feet can continue to grow in both length and width up to one full shoe size? This is due to the softening of the bones, and stretching of the foot ligaments. No wonder your feet hurt. Remember, aching feet take all of the beauty from your face. Check your size!

329
Smear? NO FEAR

For those pesky makeup mistakes, (blobs of mascara, eye shadow droppings, etc.) rather than making a mess by cleansing or rubbing and smearing even more, **take a cotton swab, dip it into your foundation and erase the mistake.** This trick also works well when your lipstick is creeping up into the lines above the lips.

Scentless

If you can't afford your favorite perfume, you can still get the effect by wearing the less expensive form, such as body splash, powder, shower gel, or deodorant.

331
In The Mix

Make your own perfumed body lotion or cream by adding a couple of drops of your signature fragrance or essential oil to a plain, unscented lotion or cream. Simply mix the two together in your hand and apply.

SAY ALOE

The gel of the Aloe Vera plant has been used as a healing agent since ancient times. To keep the burn cooling, irritation soothing, itchy skin reliever on hand, consider getting an aloe plant for your home. When an unexpected skin malady arises, simply cut a piece of a spike from the cactus like plant and smooth the fluid from the plant over the involved area for instant relief. Now doesn't that feel better?

333
Out Of The Cold

If a cold sore/fever blister suddenly comes on the scene, ice it. Putting ice on a beginning cold sore lowers the skin's metabolic rate and stops the cold sore from turning over as quickly. Another way is to bathe the blister in 3% hydrogen peroxide or rubbing alcohol (do not apply if the skin is broken). Afterwards, place a wet, cool tea bag on the area for 5 minutes. The tannic acid in the tea reduces a cold sore's inflammation.

Bedside Manner

Lips can dry out during the night, especially if you breathe through your mouth while sleeping or if the bedroom is warm and dry. To keep lips their softest, line free, and most kissable, nourish them nocturnally. *Keep some moisturizing, vitamin enriched lip balm on the nightstand.*

Scale Down Flaky Scalp

Sprinkling an antibacterial mouthwash like Listerine® is a very effective treatment for flaky scalp because it keeps the yeast level down. Mix ½ cup of water and ½ cup of mouthwash together and gently massage into the scalp after shampooing. Rinse well and then style as usual.

You can now tell the flakes to flake off.

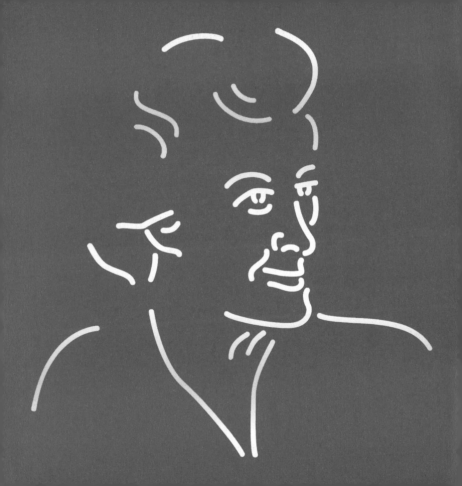

Chapter 12

Ageless

"The great thing about getting older is that you don't lose all of the other ages you have been."
Madeline L'Engle

Strike the word 'anti-aging' from your vocabulary. The word is defined as: against or in opposition to aging. It is impossible to 'anti-age'—if we are to continue living, growing, and being. *Opt instead to become ageless, which means eternal and timeless.*

YOUR FUTURE IS BRIGHT

So bright that you need to wear sunglasses and sunscreen. **Nothing ages your skin faster than exposure to the sun's rays.** Sun damage is cumulative. The past will come back to haunt you. The all day baking of youth, will appear in the form of extra wrinkles, uneven pigmentation, age spots, and maybe even potential cancer sites later on.

WORK IT!

Exercise daily. Use it or lose it. Too much sitting on the sidelines produces obesity, cardiovascular problems, stiff joints, dull hair and skin, and low energy. Be your age, but don't look it.

Never say never

Never think or say things like, "After all, I am not getting any younger" or "I am no spring chicken." Replace the negative self-talk or verbiage with positive thoughts and words such as "I am as young as I feel!" or "I am not aging, I am marinating!" Keeping a young attitude and thought process will keep you fresh and young. **Think young to remain young.**

NEVER TOO LATE!

Always remember it is never too late to make

really dramatic changes to your diet, exercise, or

beauty routine. **Never be**

complacent.

Embracing You

Whatever you do... make it an adventure.

Explore, and discover things, places, and who you are on a daily basis.

No Truer Words

Remember the word impossible is really just 'I'm possible'. Be open to new things and new ways. Reinvent yourself.

MORE THAN SKIN DEEP

True beauty and supreme agelessness is more than skin deep. *It is a style, a manner, a being and most importantly an attitude.*

Get one today!

Coming Of Age

We are living longer than ever before. In the early 1900s the average lifespan was only 46 years old. Now it is 77. And 47 years of age is the age when most of us are finally realizing success in so many areas of our lives. Celebrate everyday!

344

Never, Never Land

The term 'act your age' is not encouraging. In fact, it is an insult. Resist that limited way of thinking. Remember you are as old as you feel.

Think young—be young!

345

There is strength in numbers

Repetitions that is.

Adding a strength training session to your weekly running, cycling, or aerobics program will dramatically increase your anti-aging efforts in all of the good ways!

KNOCK OUT!

Fighting Mother Nature is good exercise. Plan to go the distance. Prepare like a professional—workout, eat right, and psyche yourself up. Remember, as Ali said, **"float like a butterfly—sting like a bee."**

Just Say No!

One of the main causes of stress is overloading our plate—with commitments that pull us in a zillion different directions. **To have lasting beauty inside and out—just say no to too many extra curricular activities.** Keep some 'me time' in your schedule—every day, not just on weekends or special occasions. Say N-O to guilt, too, if you 'can't do it all'. Remember you can still 'have it all'. Be a tad selfish for you.

348

Keep Smiling

On the average, children smile about 400 times a day while adults only smile 15! Smiling tightens the supporting skin connective tissue all around the mouth and cheeks, which helps to strengthen and maintain facial shape. **Plus, smiling sends a good feeling message to the brain making you feel better.** Say Cheese!

349

Energize
Don't Compromise

It is a myth that as we age we lose our energy.

Low energy level is usually related to poor diet,

too little exercise, and not enough sleep. **The**
surest way to optimum
energy is to eat right, move
it, and get some sleep!

WHAT'S THAT SMELL?

As we age, our sense of smell declines by as much as 50%.

To keep your nose in the know, expose yourself to various fragrances a few times a day. Mix them up, create a variety of perfumes from pungent odors to sweet florals. Enjoy scented candles to keep the nose knowing.

351

Tasteless

Since the sense of smell controls about 90% of the sense of taste, food could taste blander as the sense of smell subsides. As a result, cravings for saltier foods or more sweet treats can occur. To combat the 'bland taste', chew each bit of food more, this allows more aroma to reach your nose. It also aids in food digestion. SPICE IT UP WITH SOME EXOTIC SPICES FOR A ZIPPY YOUNG PALATE.

Supplement Insurance

Taking optimal amounts of nutritional supplements is a cornerstone and key component of a comprehensive ageless program. **The food we eat does not have enough of the nutrients that we need for optimum ageless health**. Make an appointment with an anti-aging specialist to see exactly what nutrients you need to stay your youngest.

353

Food Of The Gods

Garlic has been used since ancient times and has been proven to have anti-bacterial, anti-viral, and anti-fungal properties.

Garlic also improves the immune system, lowers cholesterol and blood pressure, and reduces chances of strokes. *Garlic is truly an all-around winner for agelessness.* One clove a day is all you need, or supplement equally.

Ageless three F's

Fruits, fish, and fiber.

Eat at least **5** servings of fruits and vegetables a day, eat more fish than meat, and incorporate light fiber into your daily diet for the most stay-young benefits.

10 Versus 20

New studies show that exercising for even just 10 minutes a day, if your schedule won't allow for 20 minutes, has the same benefits of exercising longer, provided that you do it every day. Who would not want to spare 10 minutes a day to a) live longer and b) look better? This is an-all-of-the-above answer and a real no-brainer get moving... now!

356

THE NUMBER ONE ANTI-AGER

Confidence. It is smart, sexy and sassy. Learn to shine with your confidence and not only will everyone totally believe that you are gorgeous, but younger than your years. Strut your stuff—confidently.

I Can't Hear You

Speak clearly and confidently when you talk. Inject enthusiasm into the tone of your voice rather than droning on in a dull monotone. Speak the voice of the young and vibrant, not the old and withdrawn. **It is not what you say but how you say it.**

Lip Sense

NOTHING AGES YOU FASTER THAN UNSIGHTLY STAINS ON YOUR TEETH.

Brighten your smile and teeth by using a whitening tooth polish. If that doesn't work, consult your dentist about bleaching. Have metal fillings replaced with white natural looking ones. Also flesh colored, brownish mauve, or terracotta hued lip color make teeth look whiter.

Less Is **MORE**

Go lighter rather than heavier on the makeup. Too much makeup has a way of settling into the lines and (gasp!) wrinkles, making them look more prominent. Instead opt for lighter foundations with a light defusing powder that deflects rather than reflects wrinkles. Remember the famous line from the movie *Sunset Boulevard* "Mr. DeMille I am ready for my close up!"—not pretty!

Sun Damage Is Accumulative

Sunburns are not only unattractive and dangerous, they also reflect someone who is obviously out of touch with the times. Just one sunburn can double our chances of skin cancer—even if it has been years since you've fried yourself to a crisp. **Sunburns can also weaken your immune system and your ability to battle diseases.** NOTHING is worth that—cover up.

Check it Out

INVEST IN A FULL-LENGTH MIRROR FOR YOUR BEDROOM, BATHROOM, OR CLOSET.

Use it to see how you look coming and going.

Some of the most obvious signs of aging or 'un-beauty' are seen coming from behind.

Remember to always check yours!

Funny Bone

When exfoliating, buffing, and hydrating, remember your elbows. WRINKLY, DRY AND 'ASHEN' LOOKING ELBOWS ARE A SURE SIGN OF AGING.

COMING UP ROSEMARY

Rosemary is packed with antioxidants. Use this aromatic herb to season fish, vegetables, and egg dishes. Antioxidant rich foods and seasonings are the smart answer to becoming ageless.

364

WHAT'S UP DOC?

Studies show that eating **5** carrots a week may reduce chances of having a stroke by up to **68%.** Carrots contain beta-carotene, the precursor to vitamin A. An easy way to add this healthy habit to your diet is to dice a carrot in your salad, or try adding some carrot pieces to a bowl of soup or maybe just wash and cut a carrot to carry with you for a quick snack. It is worth it, don't you think?

I GOT TO BE *Me*

When creating your own very personal style, be sure to take into account all the wonderful things you possess that make you who you are. *Dress, look, act, be, and reflect the spirit that is naturally you!* Smile, you are beautiful!

About The Author

Susie Galvez, esthetician and makeup artist, is the owner of Face Works Day Spa in Richmond, Virginia and the founder of her own skin care line. Her spa has been featured in national and consumer magazines such as *Allure*, *Cosmopolitan*, *Elle*, and *Town and Country* as well as trade publications including *Skin, Inc.*, *Dermascope*, *Day Spa*, *Salon Today*, *Nails Plus*, *Nails*, *Spa Management*, and *Les Nouvelles Esthetiques* among others. In April 2002, The Day Spa Association recognized Face Works as one of only twelve fully accredited day spas in North America out of over one thousand members.

Ms. Galvez's first book *"InSPArations"* is an industry success. The book has been featured in spa industry magazines internationally. In addition to speaking at international spa conventions, Susie is a regular contributor to beauty publications. She is also a television and radio spokesperson for the beauty industry.

Special Appreciation

"Each friend represents a world in us, a world possibly not born until they arrive, and it is only by this meeting that a new world is born." Anais Nin

This book could not have been completed without the unwavering support and love from my very special friends. Thank you to:

Jody Allen, doctoral candidate, whose command of the English language and proof-reading skills were put to the test on this manuscript but who was always gentle in how she suggested 'perhaps a better way to say it.' And she was right.

Dennis Michael Stredney, graphic designer, who 'gets it' each and every time a word or idea is thrown at him and turns my words into art.